I Get It!
Building Social Thinking® and Reading Comprehension Through Book Chats

by Audra Jensen, M.Ed., BCBA

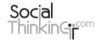

Social Thinking Publishing, San Jose, California
www.socialthinking.com

I Get It! Building Social Thinking® and Reading Comprehension Through Book Chats

Audra Jensen, M.Ed., BCBA

Book images reprinted with permission of respective publishers. Norman Rockwell paintings reprinted with permission of Norman Rockwell Museum and The Rockwell Family Agency.

Edited by Sandra Horwich, Sandra Horwich and Associates, Inc., www.shorwich.com
Layout and Cover Design by Elizabeth Blacker
Cover image by Design Pics/Leah Warkentin, gettyimages.com

Library of Congress Control Number: 2011937407
Social Thinking Publishing

ISBN: 978-1-936943-01-2
Social Thinking Publishing
San Jose, California

Social Thinking Publishing
3031 Tisch Way #800
San Jose, CA 95128
Toll-free Phone: (877) 464-9278
Fax: (408) 557-8594

This book is printed and bound in Michigan by Thomson-Shore, Inc.

Books can be ordered online at www.socialthinking.com.

This is dedicated to Audra Margaret Jensen, the Junior. While this book technically has nothing to do with you, your patience and enduring love of your sometimes preoccupied mother deserves more than a little dedication in the beginning of a book. You are a wonderful person, a patient sister (at least try to be!), a good Social Thinking group peer, and the daughter I could never dream of until you came along. You enrich my life.

Contents

||||||||||||||||||||||||||||||||||||||||||||||||||||||||||||||||||||||||||||||||||||||||||||||||||||||||||||||||||||||||||||

Foreword

|||||||||||||||||||||||||||||||||||||||||||||||||||||||||||||||||||||||||||||||||||||||||||||||||||||||||||||||||||||||||||||||||||||

By Michelle Garcia Winner

In 1995 I began to work as a speech language pathologist (SLP) for the Campbell Union High School District in San Jose, California. Unclear as to the role of an SLP with high school age students, I bought a book on communication disorders and learning disabilities. This was before implementation of No Child Left Behind, after which educators became focused on how to ensure that all students, including our special education students, achieved mastery of their coursework as it correlates to educational standards. In 1995, I attempted to assess students' learning and communication needs to help them learn concepts and skills to ultimately better manage in society. Most of the students I worked with were also recognized as having learning disabilities, which meant they were taught the Language Arts curriculum in the Resource classroom (a special education classroom) on campus; some were mainstreamed for this subject but most were not. To better comprehend the communication and learning demands on my students across the school day, I decided to deepen my understanding of the core curriculum being taught in their classrooms. To do this, I spent a significant amount of time in the classrooms themselves exploring the academic load, observing how my students engaged with the coursework, and seeing how they were being taught. In the meantime, the Individualized Education Program (IEP) goals that had been previously written for my students, the goals I was to help my students reach, mostly related to learning better conversation and problem solving skills.

As I observed my students in class, on campus, and in my sessions, and spoke to their parents and teachers, I began to understand my students had deeper learning needs than those reported in their IEPs. Their challenges with processing instructions, interpreting the meaning of information conveyed through social interaction, inferencing and abstracting, absorbing the gist of a message or curriculum, taking perspectives of people in context, and knowing when and how to initiate communication, led me to create the ILAUGH Model of Social Cognition (Winner, 2000). With this evidence-based model, I attempted to explain to school educational personnel, administrators, parents, and ancillary clinicians the importance of observing the connections among social knowledge, social skills, and the ability to interpret and respond accurately to aspects of the students' curriculum that require social knowledge, such as reading comprehension of literature, written expression of ideas, and even organizational skills. At the same time, I was exploring treatment strategies to help my students learn better coping skills for the steadily increasing social and academic demands they faced.

The teachers and administrators with whom I worked closely became increasingly interested in talking to me about the problems they observed in their classrooms. The more they shared, the clearer it became: reading comprehension of literature is not simply about being able to read words and sentences fluently. It is also about being able to explore the stories' social contexts, the characters' perspectives, and their emotions. Doing so allows the reader to understand the source of the problems a character experiences and to predict what a character might do next. To actively read for meaning necessitates one to foreshadow upcoming events, social dilemmas, and possible solutions. This requires the development of problem solving skills using key aspects of social knowledge—it requires most of the skills discussed in the ILAUGH Model.

As I gradually came to this realization, I began to teach differently. Gone were the days of treating classroom material as separate from social knowledge and related social interactions. Instead, I carefully observed students. If they could not take a person's perspective when they were expected to socially relate to that person, I could find evidence that the same students were not able to take perspective of the characters they were reading about in their classrooms. From my standpoint, the relationship between literature and social skills became highly aligned and entwined. Yet little was written about this in the research, and teachers were given virtually no information that would help them teach deeper social learning concepts even in the special education classrooms.

Fast forward to 2011; emerging from these formative experiences, Social Thinking® has now become a treatment model that has two dimensions. One dimension is to instruct educational professionals, counselors, OTs, and parents to recognize the multifaceted issues that impact social relations and curriculum development and to identify the concepts and skills students need to develop for adult life based on a student's social cognitive learning strengths and weaknesses. The other dimension involves creating a multitude of treatment strategies to help our students have a better chance at learning social cognitive information, which in turn will aid them in becoming more competent participants within events that require astute social knowledge. Helping adult caregivers as well as students to understand the link between their social behaviors (social skills) and reading comprehension has been a major campaign.

Enter Audra Jensen. In 2008, she presented at my first annual International Social Thinking Providers Conference. Audra, a BCBA by training and a parent of a child on the autism spectrum, demonstrated the strategies she was creating. These involved using stories with strong visual pictures to help our students recognize and explore social knowledge within the pages of a book and relate those experiences back to their own personal social interactions. In doing this, she was able to provide a motivating context through which the students could explicitly explore, explain, and experience the messages implied in the books they read. This proved to be a strong tool that encourages our students to take their time to learn more about social information. I immediately asked Audra if she would consider writing a book to share her teachings with others. Audra readily agreed—this sounded simple at the time. After all, she had already created many of the treatment ideas and was teaching how to take our Social Thinking vocabulary and concepts (such as "thinking with your eyes," "Is their body in the group?," and "Did that make you have a weird thought or a good thought?") and teach them across the social academic divide. How hard could it be to write that all down? It turns out that it takes a significant amount of time to clearly express concepts and ideas in book form. Along the way, Audra did a stellar job pulling together a solid literature review to present the relationships between academic learning, research, and social learning. For those astute followers of strategies developed to better teach Social Thinking, she instructs how this book elaborates upon the core ideas. Most importantly, she presents with great clarity an organized approach by detailing specific books to teach specific concepts while explaining how to foster a deeper interpersonal relationship with students as they engage in the process. In addition, she provides a large range of goal ideas teachers and clinicians can use in an IEP to encourage this more holistic teaching technique. In a nutshell, she has created a tool that expands the wingspan of teaching Social Thinking into an elementary child's home and school day through the use of books. How cool is that?

Introduction

||||||||||||||||||||||||||||||||||||||||||||||||||||||||||||||||||||||||||||||||||||||||||||||||||||||||||||||||||

Our Story

In 1997, my husband and I were blessed with a perfectly healthy baby boy. How naively happy we were! As new parents, we didn't think much past the next diaper change, let alone far into the future. When our son was diagnosed with autism at the age of two, our lives changed. We had a mission beyond what we anticipated when we started a family.

Our son had hyperlexia in addition to autism, which meant that he spontaneously learned to read at a very young age (two years old). Because of his interest in the written word, we modified all our therapies to take advantage of this tremendous skill. We decorated our home with index cards to teach him the names of objects around him, used books as reinforcers and teaching tools, and provided him with noisy learning toys. His amazing progress was due in large part to his keen intellect and ability to learn through the written word.

What I didn't understand at the time was that he was already exhibiting classic social thinking deficits that would later inhibit his social learning *and* reading comprehension. Oh, he could *read*. He read his first word before two, and by two-and-a-half could easily read at the second grade level although he had received almost no direct instruction. However, he was simply reading the words, breaking the code. He did not understand them. He could read the words "I want a cookie" but have no idea that if he said the phrase he could be requesting a cookie from a communicative partner. Some professionals hypothesized that his reading comprehension would improve as his language did. Certainly, as his language skills increased, his ability to understand what he read got better as well. But, even when he could understand the meaning behind a sentence, he would be just as likely to "talk to the cosmos" (as we liked to say), expecting to get a cookie, as to direct his words *to* someone. It became clear to me that improvement in his reading comprehension depended less on improvement in his language comprehension and more on his ability to learn socially. For example, he could read the words in *Harry Potter* at about the age of three. He could understand the sentence structure and paragraphs and what the words *said* by about the age of eight, but he didn't *understand* and *enjoy* the story until he was about ten. I knew this was when he had gained the reading comprehension skills for the book because it was at that age that he quickly devoured all the books in the series. It was also at about that time that he became a pretty good *social thinker*. When he started to learn social thinking, I began to understand the correlation between his reading comprehension ability and his social ability.

My purpose in writing this book was twofold. I wanted to look at and analyze the research available on reading comprehension and develop my own thoughts about how it relates to social thinking. In addition, I wanted to share a technique I developed in my work with students with social cognitive difficulties (particularly autism and Asperger's Syndrome). This technique involves using children's literature to teach social thinking and to develop reading comprehension. Chapter 1 looks at social thinking and reading comprehension and the recent research in the field. Chapters 2 and 3 present Michelle Garcia Winner's framework for Social Thinking. Chapter 4 contains the technique I call the Book Chat that makes use of children's literature, often picture books, to teach social thinking. Chapter 5 speaks to current educational standards and reading comprehension strategies most often employed in the classroom. Chapters 6 through 21 provide examples of Book Chat literature and suggestions for combining social thinking and reading comprehension strategies. Chapter 22 has a list of possible goals that merge social thinking and reading comprehension strategies for use by educators or other professionals.

1

Reading Comprehension and Students with Social Cognitive Disorders

||||||||||||||||||||||||||||||||||||||||||||||||||||||||||||||||||||||||||||||||||||||||||||||||||||||||||||||||||||||||||||||||||||||||||||

Perspective Taking and Social Cognitive Disorders

Social referencing occurs in babies as young as nine months old (Franco, 1997; Walden & Ogan, 1988). This entails using eyes to show thinking—referencing a partner to see what he or she is seeing and thinking about. This means looking at facial expressions and body language and using that information to decipher the social world. Babies are already thinking with their eyes. From there, children begin to develop Theory of Mind—the ability to understand that one's thoughts, emotions, and reactions differ from those of the people around them (Baron-Cohen, Leslie, & Frith, 1985). Perspective taking (a step beyond Theory of Mind in which empathy takes a more active role) is the process of understanding differing thoughts and emotions and then changing behavior in accordance with that knowledge. Selman (1999) identified stages typically-developing children go through. These begin with a child being aware that his or her thoughts and emotions are different than those of other individuals. That awareness influences that child's behavior. Children then become more objective in analyzing those interactions. Finally they develop the awareness that even understanding and changing behavior doesn't always create complete understanding and that different social groups create their own social rules. It's a long and complicated process.

Students with social cognitive disorders are weak in the development of these perspective taking skills. Often, they are not as good as their peers at predicting what someone else is thinking and adjusting their own thoughts and behavior accordingly. That ability to predict and adjust is a vital social learning concept that impacts not only students' social development but also their ability to relate to social lessons embedded in academic curricula. By the time most children start decoding literature for comprehension, they have enough social knowledge and related social relationship practice to make sense of what the characters in a book are thinking and doing. However, students with social thinking difficulties are often missing that comprehension—their social software doesn't run well. Some students barely understand the concept that others *have* thoughts and emotions separate from their own, while other students may simply be inefficient in processing the load of all this information. These students may interpret the information correctly and react appropriately, but if they don't do it quickly enough, their peers have moved on, and they are left with an unsuccessful interaction. Whether the cause is an inability to make appropriate social observations or they are simply too slow in processing to do it efficiently, the result is the same. They are left with a series of what they consider social "failures." These social breakdowns stack up, forming a pattern, causing anxiety and a feeling of inadequacy. At that point, students are dealing not only with core difficulties of interactions but also with a feeling that they are not good at it anyway, so why try? Anxiety increases, and cognitive access to competencies decreases—a downward spiral.

This same pattern may occur when students read. Students with social cognitive disorders may read about a social interaction and struggle to understand it while the group or teacher has moved on. As a result, students are left behind, cultivating feelings of failure and anxiety. After a while, students often begin to dislike reading because they have difficulty understanding the concepts that seem basic to their typically-developing classroom peers.

Many students with social cognitive disorders have test scores that reveal strong academic and language skills, but such scores can be misleading. Educators or professionals may erroneously assume that reading comprehension is not a concern if the students have high cognitive skills, can decode (read the words), and are able to answer questions about what they read. Most assessments, especially in the formative years, measure decoding and factual information only. By these measures, students with high cognitive ability but social deficits may score well and get passed on year after year without intervention. While these students *can* decode well, often well above grade level, they fall short when it comes to interpreting literature. They can often answer questions that ask who, where, when, and what: "Where did the boys go after they found the note?," "What did the girl do when she got home from school?," or "Where did the boy find the lost shoe?" However, if asked *why* the boys went to the old man's house when they read the note, what made them *think* the girl was going to change out of her clothes when she got home, or what in the story led them to *believe* that the shoe was still at the bus stop, they struggle to find the correct answer. Students with social cognitive difficulties find it problematic to put themselves into a story, engage with the characters, and understand perspectives and how different people and situations affect each other and their environment. They have difficulty comprehending implicit information such as predictions and inferences, understanding emotional responses, interpreting motives, and identifying the main idea. These are the same issues they have in their daily social communicative interactions and social interpretations. If they can't do it in person, it would make sense that they would find it difficult to cognitively understand and respond to the same concepts when presented in the pages of a book.

Reading Comprehension Research

Written Language versus Spoken Language

Many components of language comprehension contribute to successful reading comprehension. Language comprehension requires competence in phonology, semantics, syntax, and pragmatics (Bishop, 1997). These components also influence the understanding of written language, but the data is mixed on the extent of that influence. Vocabulary has a clear correlation between spoken and written language. Lack of early word identification and phonological skills does limit reading comprehension, but that influence diminishes with age and reading progress.

Language comprehension contributes to reading comprehension; however, reading comprehension is more than simple decoding of words. Written language is much different than spoken language. Written language is not merely speech written down on paper but makes use of language in ways that may be unfamiliar to the reader whether it uses more formal wording, different vocabulary, or different syntactic schema (Cunningham, 2005; Garton & Pratt, 1998; Reid, 1970, 1983). In addition to the differences in language and syntax, two significant other differences make written language more difficult to fully understand for students with social cognitive impairments. First, written language is displaced from the student's reality. It's not happening right now, so it takes a level of forethought and the ability to synthesize information. Second, written language requires that the reader move forward without explicit clarification (Garton & Pratt, 1998). In spoken language, a listener can stop the speaker and ask for clarification, whereas a reader cannot do this with an author. Thus, even when students progress in their listening comprehension, their reading comprehension may still lag behind (Cain & Oakhill, 2007). This differs significantly from the "simple view" of reading presented by Gough and colleagues (1986), which asserted that an individual's reading comprehension would develop to the same level as listening comprehension as long as word decoding was strong.

Reading Comprehension

So, what *does* reading comprehension depend on? In their review of the research literature, Oakhill and Cain (2007) identify three distinct predictors of reading comprehension: the ability to answer inferential questions, the ability to monitor comprehension (metacognition), and the capacity to understand story structure. Generally, the ability to make inferences develops with age (Barnes, Dennis, & Haefele-Kalvaitis, 1996). If it doesn't, students struggle to comprehend written language. To successfully understand text, students have to analyze what information is given, use their own general knowledge to fill in missing details, and then synthesize that information to construct appropriate outcomes. This entails an ability to analyze whether their hypotheses are correct or false and then make changes as necessary, actions that require students to use higher-level metacognition. If students make an incorrect inference, they must discern it and adjust accordingly. In addition, if students do *not* comprehend a passage, they must *recognize* that shortfall before they can even make the necessary adjustments. How complicated!

In addition to self-monitoring and inferencing, the knowledge of story structure has been shown to be an important predictor of reading comprehension (Cain & Oakhill, 2007; Trabasso & Nickels, 1992; Perfetti, 1994). Cain and Oakhill (2003b and 2007) report that measuring the comprehension of story structure is the strongest predictor of later comprehension between the ages of seven and ten. Trabasso and Nickels (1992) conclude that the text connections are usually the most crucial to understanding the overall theme of text and to integrating information. The ability to understand the flow of a story—the structure and important elements—can be assessed even before students begin reading. In fact, the comprehension of aural stories (stories told to or read to the student) is highly correlated with later reading comprehension (Kendeou et al., 2006; Kendeou, van den Broek, White & Lynch, 2007; van den Broek et al., 2005).

Relationship Between Decoding and Comprehending

Cain and Oakhill (2007) find that the widely held view that reading comprehension develops once decoding is in place is inconsistent with current research. Although decoding and comprehension often occur in relation to one another, there is a group of readers who develop word and sentence decoding while being behind in reading comprehension. These students are referred to as having *specific comprehension deficit* or are described as "poor comprehenders." Cain, Oakhill, and Lemmon (2004) point out that "good and poor comprehenders who are matched for knowledge of written and spoken word meanings can differ on standardized measures of reading comprehension."

There are also students who learn to read spontaneously and precociously or without direct instruction but whose comprehension lags far behind. These are students with *hyperlexia*, a term first coined by Silberberg and Silberberg in 1967 to describe individuals whose word decoding ability is significantly higher than their reading comprehension and whose early and advanced reading abilities stand in stark contrast to other developmental delays. Students with early, precocious reading abilities but no developmental delays are not considered hyperlexic, merely advanced readers. Approximately 5-10% of students with autism spectrum disorders show evidence of hyperlexia (Aaron, 1989; Burd & Kerbeshian, 1985; Burd, Kerbeshian & Fisher, 1985; Grigorenko, Klin, Pauls, Senft, Hooper & Volkmar, 2002). Hyperlexia is not a formal medical diagnosis; it is used to describe the symptoms of high decoding and low comprehension combined with developmental delays (different than being a "poor comprehender"). However, with 5-10% of students with autism displaying such contrasting skills, it's important to take note of it.

A common method of evaluating students' reading in elementary school is with the use of fluency measures (how fast a student reads). While this is a great assessment tool for word decoding and comprehension that stem merely from decoding deficits, fluency is not necessarily a valid measure of reading comprehension when decoding is not the problem (Paris, Carpenter, Pairs & Hamilton, 2005). In one study, reading fluency was not a reliable measure of overall reading competence for students either with high-functioning autism or students with high-functioning autism with evidence of hyperlexia. In fact, students with hyperlexia had extremely diverse fluency and comprehension measure scores (Jensen, 2006). So although fluency measures may be one way to assess reading competence in many students, it may not be a reliable measure for students with autism.

Reading Comprehension in Children with Autism Spectrum Disorders

Students on the autism spectrum are one of the most prevalent groups of students with social cognitive disorders. Even those with high cognitive abilities and who are considered "high-functioning" show distinctive difficulties in reading (Minshew et al., 1994; Happe, 1997; Snowling & Frith, 1986). The evidence that they struggle with reading comprehension is extensive. For example, Nation et al. (2006) studied 41 children with autism spectrum disorders and found that text reading accuracy was within normal ranges, but reading comprehension was impaired. Asberg (2009) states that in addition to reading comprehension deficiencies being a common thread among children with autism spectrum disorders, their discourse-level comprehension is more impaired than expected given their nonverbal cognitive skills. This is no surprise for those of us working in the field with these students.

To understand text, skilled readers must integrate current information with background knowledge and synthesize it to analyze the meaning of text. For students on the autism spectrum, switching attention between different tasks may be problematic (Courchesne et al., 1994; Plaisted, 1999; Shah & Frith, 1993). Therefore, students might also struggle with integrating background knowledge to understand the meaning of a text. In contrast, skilled readers make use of prior knowledge to gain reading comprehension (Pressley & Afflerbach, 1995), which is not the case for students with autism (Snowling & Frith, 1986; Wahlberg & Magliano, 2004). Wahlberg's study found that students with autism could "access" background information; they just didn't apply it to interpret information accurately. Not only do students with autism have trouble applying background information, when dealing with social situations, the background information itself may be inaccurate. In these cases, even if students correctly apply their background knowledge, they can still have problems with comprehension because their understanding of that knowledge is inaccurate. It's a two-pronged problem that requires multiple interventions, which brings us to the role of social knowledge in reading comprehension.

What Role Does Social Knowledge Play?

In their review of recent reading research, Paris and Hamilton conclude that "decoding is necessary but not sufficient for comprehension" (2009, 33). Although much of the research on reading comprehension supports that comprehension does not solely depend on decoding, the second factor attributed to reading comprehension is typically language comprehension (Gough & Tunmer, 1986; LaBerge & Samuels, 1974; Stahl & Heibert, 2005; Stahl, Kuh & Pickle, 1999). There is little to differentiate basic language skills from pragmatic language skills when it comes to reading comprehension. Much of the research has been on vocabulary and syntax as measures of language ability (Paris & Hamilton, 2009). In their review of the literature, Paris and Hamilton state, "It is unclear how children develop skills needed to construct text base and situation models and how to integrate their previous knowledge with the constructed representation" (2009, 36). Frith and Snowling (1983) observe that students with high-functioning autism lack understanding of the semantics of sentences. In a study using cloze tasks, students selected words that were syntactically (or grammatically) appropriate but not necessarily semantically appropriate to have the sentences make social sense.

In the past, there has been limited research on the role of social knowledge in reading comprehension. However, Kintsch (1998) presented the Construction-Integration (CI) model of reading that is beginning to take hold in the research. The CI model states that the reader's ability to make inferences and go beyond the text base is required for skilled comprehension. This requires connecting content to previous experience and knowledge and an ability to activate relevant schemata, which are small containers in which we deposit our knowledge of certain subjects and experiences (Anderson & Pearson, 1984; Rumelhart, 1994). Making inferences requires readers to look at a variety of elements (both explicit

7

and implicit) and relate that information to background knowledge. This is vital to reading comprehension (Oakhill, Yuill & Parkin, 1986; Cain & Oakhill, 1999; Oakhill, Cain & Bryan, 2003; Laing & Kamhi, 2002). In addition, teaching students *how* to make inferences has been shown to improve their reading comprehension (McGee & Johnson, 2003; Yuill & Oakhill, 1988; Reutzel & Hollingsworth, 1988; Carr, Dewitz & Patberg, 1983; Vidal-Abarca, Martinez & Gilabert, 2000). Goldstein et al. (1994) found that reading comprehension for students with high-functioning autism was similar to IQ-matched controls; for adolescents, however, reading comprehension was lower than controls, possibly reflecting the greater inferential demands of age-normed tests for older students.

This takes into account an ability to infer beyond what the text directly states, which takes a level of social awareness. Westby (2008) states that, "[i]f children do not understand emotionality and temporal cause-effect relationships in social situations, they will not be able to use such knowledge . . . for text comprehension." Today most contemporary theories tell us that reading comprehension requires understanding of others' points of view, related emotional responses, and monitoring of characters' intentions (Pelletier & Astington, 2004; Bruner, 1986). Theory of Mind and the ability to understand another's perspective depend on social understanding, which is acquired through conversation and interaction with others (Garfield, Peterson & Perry, 2001). Theory of Mind is necessary to comprehend what characters are thinking and why they are behaving in a certain way. Perspective taking is a must not only to *know* what characters are thinking but to know *why* they are thinking that way and what might happen in the future based on the many complexities of social interactions. Social knowledge is essential.

Students with social cognitive challenges are missing the exact thing that current research has neglected to look at in depth. For example, Rathvon (2004) lists ten components of reading and The National Reading Panel (2000) identifies five components of reading that include a variety of word reading skills as well as language and vocabulary; however, neither list mentions social knowledge or related abilities. "Comprehension" is stated as a component in each list as a standalone item. How big of a role does social knowledge play in reading comprehension? Each year that more students come through my clinic with associated social knowledge and reading comprehension challenges, the more convinced I am that the two are strongly correlated, but more research is needed.

Westby (2004) points out that to be a skilled reader, students must have knowledge about what is being read and be able to relate information from their own experiences to the present text. However, if students have not had successful social interactions or do not interpret the social world accurately, they cannot apply that knowledge when reading. Paris and Hamilton (2009) summarize their research by suggesting guidelines to help young readers develop good comprehension, the first being "teach background knowledge." Although they refer to concepts and themes in the literature, I suggest it also means teaching social thinking to provide students with *social* background knowledge.

The Shifting Trend from Pure Behaviorism to Cognitive Strategy Instruction

Radical behaviorism asserts that all behavior is environmentally controlled and discounts, at least to some degree, the role of private events or thought processes. This view was prevalent in the field of psychology for 50 years. At that point, cognitive psychologists began to look at the role of the mind in the existence of behavior. Today's behaviorism still focuses on operant conditioning where the environment is manipulated in such a way that it causes a behavior to be more likely to increase or decrease in the future. Most professionals in the field of behavior analysis (myself included) recognize, and the research supports, the idea that changing the environment is highly effective in changing behavior. If students are motivated by goldfish crackers, they will be more likely to do what you ask if they know they will get some for their correct performance. If they don't like the crackers, they will be less likely to engage in the behavior you seek if they don't want to do it. However, most behaviorists recognize that cognitive processes and states of being have an influence on behavior. If those students have already had a big bag of goldfish, they may be less likely to engage in a desired behavior to get one. They're sick of them! On the other hand, if they're hungry and haven't eaten in a while, they will be more likely to engage in that behavior to get the crackers. In addition, if by eating goldfish crackers, students expect to be teased by their peers and they care about being teased by peers, they will also be less likely to engage in the desired behavior to get the crackers even if they're hungry and want some. Their "mind" state has an influence on behavior.

In recent decades, traditional behavior therapy has merged with cognitive therapy to produce cognitive behavior therapy or CBT. This is a form of treatment in which "thinking" has a huge role in shaping behavior. Typically with CBT, patients understand what behaviors they want to change, why they want to change them, and have some power over controlling them for the sake of internal gratification, social acceptance, or goal reaching. Obviously, this language based-metacognitive technique is not effective for cognitively-impaired, limited language students. This method of teaching does not play to their strengths. However, it can be ideal for students who are able to learn by developing insight into their own and others' perspective taking and related social emotional behaviors. This can be done through language-based discussion and by developing better observational skills related to the intricacies of the social world.

In terms of reading comprehension, cognitive strategies and instruction have only recently made their way into education. *Cognitive strategies* are the activities needed for handling incoming information and *metacognitive strategies* are activities needed for monitoring and evaluating the understanding of that information (Greeno, Collins & Resnick, 1996; van Dijk & Kintsch, 1983). A cognitive strategy is what your mind has to *do* to accomplish a cognitive goal. For example, as they read, skilled readers ask questions to themselves about *what* they are reading and if it is making sense. To teach this, teachers may model this strategy by reading a text selection in front of the class, pausing throughout to ask thinking questions out loud ("Hmmm, I wonder why she went back to the bus stop."). They may even write questions on Post-It notes to help the class visualize the thought process. (Cris Tovani's *I Read it, But I Don't Get It* is a great resource to learn how to teach strategies to struggling reading comprehension students.) That is one strategy. A metacognitive strategy is how your mind assesses its own performance in accomplishing that goal. If skilled readers recognize that their own mental questions are not fixing comprehension deficiencies, they can switch to another strategy. They may ask questions of a friend who is reading the same book or look up unfamiliar words in a dictionary. They constantly evaluate whether what they are doing is moving them forward in comprehending the text, looking at how to make the reading enjoyable and informative for themselves. *Metacognition* means being familiar with particular strategies and knowing when and how to use them.

Social Thinking® and Reading Comprehension

While cognitive and metacognitive strategies are taking hold in reading comprehension instruction, understanding the use of social cognition as it relates to reading comprehension is in its infancy. Winner (2007) describes how normal social development and social thinking snowball in sophistication as students enter their upper years of elementary school and continues escalating throughout the school years. Not coincidentally, the language arts curriculum (particularly with regards to interpreting fiction) also increases in the nuance and sophistication students need to understand the thoughts and minds of the characters. As both social and academic demands grow, it is common to find that students with social cognitive difficulties have greater challenges with reading comprehension regardless of their ability to decode the text. Challs's (1967, 1996) developmental model of reading is well known and accepted in the education community. In the fourth stage, students go from "learning to read" to "reading to learn"; this typically occurs between fourth and eighth grades. By then, typically-developing students have a solid foundation for interpreting, analyzing, and succeeding in the social world. Students with social cognition deficits may have been succeeding in their "learning to read" years of school (kindergarten to second grade) but have had few successes in the social world. Thus, when asked to "read to learn" and analyze social situations in literature, they are behind their peers. During these grades (typically between fourth and eighth grade), a shift occurs in which reading to learn becomes a part of every academic subject. Students with social cognitive difficulties not only fall behind in reading comprehension but also in other subjects such as social studies and history that require understanding of motives and intentions of individuals in history.

We often *assume* students are capable of social thought if they appear intelligent based on formal testing and if they have developed the ability to use language conversationally. When students struggle with social interpretations, we often *assume* they have behavior or attention problems even though the cause may be an entirely different and often overlooked one—weak social thinking. By teaching social thinking, we support emerging literacy and written expression and social relatedness as well. Reading comprehension is not an island unto itself—it is an active part of our social functioning. Teaching social thinking in real life and through literature not only helps students improve reading comprehension but also helps them develop competent and successful social interactions.

The rest of this book provides you with ideas for how to further explore these concepts and for books you can use to help focus specific lessons and teachings. The work of Maryellen Rooney Moreau is also highly recommended. She has developed a method for teaching social emotional critical thinking as it integrates into multiple other aspects of knowledge that need to be processed and considered to interpret social situations, including those conveyed though reading comprehension of literature. Moreau's technique, which is called Story Grammar Marker®, is an evidence-based multisensory technique (see References) that meshes well with Social Thinking lessons.

2

The ILAUGH Model of Social Thinking

||||||||||||||||||||||||||||||||||||||||||||||||||||||||||||||||||||||||||||||||||||||||||||||||||||||||||||||||||||||

Social Thinking Learning Challenges

Whether we use the term *theory of mind, mind-blindness,* or the related and more complex term, *perspective taking,* we are talking about similar concepts: the ability (or inability) to recognize and respond to the feelings and thoughts of others as different from our own. In the case of perspective taking, this means being able to understand the main idea of any social moment by integrating multiple complex sets of information while discerning that our thoughts and feelings are separate from what we perceive *others* think and feel in any situation. Those with social cognitive disorders, such as autism spectrum disorders, nonverbal learning disorder (NVLD), attention deficit disorder, and the like, may not identify how their behavior affects people around them. They may have difficulty identifying the intentions of others and don't consider that others try to read their intentions and related emotions, making it hard for each person in a situation to engage in social interpretation and possibly social reciprocity.

The ILAUGH Model of Social Thinking

Michelle Garcia Winner is a speech language pathologist with an interest in social learning challenges who has worked with clients for more than 20 years. Since 1995, she has focused on the development of treatment ideas for helping students with near normal to far above normal verbal intelligence learn social thinking and related social skills. Winner created the ILAUGH Model of Social Thinking (2000) to summarize different aspects of research findings as they relate to these students' unique learning challenges. The ILAUGH Model provides a framework for better understanding of how social awareness and social learning impact not only a person's development of social skills but also one's ability to fully participate in curricula, such as reading comprehension, that also require social thinking. The following table summarizes the ILAUGH model and also includes examples from my experience at our clinic.

ILAUGH Model and Examples

		Definition
I	Initiation of Language	Initiation of language is the ability to use one's language skills to seek assistance or information. A student's ability to talk about his or her own topics of interest can be in sharp contrast to how that student communicates when in need of assistance. Students with social cognitive deficits often have difficulty asking for help, seeking clarification, and initiating appropriate social entrance and exit with other people.
L	Listening with Eyes and Brain	Most persons with social cognitive deficits have difficulty with auditory comprehension. Listening, however, requires more than just taking in the auditory information. It also requires the person to integrate information he or she sees in the context along with the nonverbal cues of the other people in the group to fully interpret the spoken or unspoken message. Classrooms depend heavily on having all students attend nonverbally to the expectations in the classroom. Thus, being a "good listener" includes attending to the verbal and nonverbal cues.
A	Abstract and Inferential Language	Communicative comprehension requires both literal and figurative interpretations. Four steps of clues help to interpret abstract communication: the listener's understanding of who the speaker is and his/her motive for communicating, in what context the message is being shared, the literal words used, as well as the nonverbal ways in which the message is coded along with the related physical gestures also used to relay the message. Thus, abstract and inferential meaning is often carried subtly through verbal and nonverbal means of communication along with social knowledge of the people and situation. This skill begins to develop in the preschool years and continues across our school years as the messages we are to interpret both socially and academically become more abstract. Interpretation depends in part on one's ability to "make a smart guess"; it also depends on one's ability to take the perspective of another. Abstract and inferential language interpretation is a major part of our language arts, social studies, and science curricula. It is also a skill set heavily applied in play and conversation.
U	Understanding Perspective	This is the ability to understand the emotions, thoughts, beliefs, experiences, motives, intentions, and personality of yourself as well as of others. Students begin to intuitively acquire this skill in early development. Neurotypical students have acquired a solid foundation in this ability between the ages of four to six as they learn to begin to manipulate and understand other people's minds. Children continue to refine their knowledge of others' minds across their lives. The ability to take perspective is key to participation in any type of group (social or academic) as well as to interpreting information that requires understanding of other people's minds, such as reading comprehension, history, social studies, etc. It is also key to formulating clear written expression. Weakness in perspective taking is a significant part of the diagnosis of social cognitive deficits.

eal examples	Examples of social behavioral challenges	Examples of how it impacts reading comprehension
group of boys are standing around lking about going to a movie this eekend. **Sam, age 14,** would like to join em, so he walks right up to them and arts talking about the weather vane he ade that weekend.	Difficulty knowing how to appropriately initiate a social interaction	Inability to recognize if a character made an appropriate initiation and how it was received by the social partners
a social group, **Ryan, age 8,** comes in few minutes late. Everyone in the group sitting in a circle, reading a book. yan does not pay attention to the group havior, and instead comes in and kes out the balls used for movement tivities and begins bouncing one. **nily, age 4,** is looking for her favorite y. Her mom tries to tell her where it is rough pointing and facial expressions. nily begins to search by going in the rection of the point but does not look ck to see what her mom is looking at/ inking about and is not able to find e toy.	Difficulty interpreting body language or simply an awareness of body language	Challenge in understanding the written description of nonverbal social interactions and how to interpret them.
idan, age 11, tells Caleb that his mom cooking ELEPHANT for dinner night. He does so with a serious face d voice tone. Caleb says that he doesn't ce elephant. Norman Rockwell painting is shown to **group of 12-year-old boys.** It depicts group of half-naked boys whose hair is et carrying their clothes, running away, d looking over their shoulders. There a sign that says "No Swimming" in e background. When asked what they ink happened, Jason responds that ey are running to the swimming pool.	Difficulty making "smart guesses" through synthesizing verbal and nonverbal clues	Not being able to make inferences, weak at interpreting idioms, sarcasm, metaphors, analogies, and indirect communication to anticipate what the characters are doing and thinking and how this information impacts the story line.
yce, age 10, loves trains. He will talk anyone about trains. In fact, he will ntinue to talk about trains even when e person he is talking to is not looking him, is yawning, and even turning his her back. **ckie, age 7,** gets frustrated in class d throws herself on the ground. She is mpletely unaware that the kids around r are having "weird or uncomfortable oughts" about her behavior and will be s likely to want to play with her at recess.	Talking about a preferred topic without appearing to be aware of the interest of the other person in the topic	Taking the perspective of the characters in the book and thinking about what the characters are thinking and feeling. Understanding how a character's behavior impacts other characters in the story. Possibly being less able to read the intentions of the character.

Definition

G	Gestalt Processing/ Getting the Big Picture	Information is conveyed through concepts and not just facts. When participating in a conversation, the participants intuitively should determine the underlying concepts being discussed. When reading, one has to follow the overall meaning (concept) rather than just collect a series of facts. Conceptual processing is another key component to understanding social and academic information. Furthermore, difficulty with organizational strategies is born from problems with conceptual processing. This skill, like all others above, is an executive function task. Weaknesses in the development of this skill can greatly impact one's ability to formulate written expression, summarize reading passages, and manage one's homework load.

H	Humor and Human Relatedness	Most students have a very good sense of humor, but they feel anxious since they miss many of the subtle cues that help them to understand how to participate successfully with others. It is important for educators/parents to work compassionately and with humor to help minimize the anxiety the children are experiencing. At the same time, many students use humor inappropriately, and direct lessons about this topic are often called for.
		Human relatedness is at the heart of social interaction. While virtually all students with social cognitive disorders desire some form of social interaction, they have difficulty relating to others' minds, emotions, and needs; working at developing a social relationship with you is a prerequisite to the child being available for social learning.

When I taught special education (students with high-functioning autism and Asperger's), I saw a trend. Inevitably, even students with test scores that measured high cognitive and academic abilities struggled with reading comprehension, math problem solving, and writing content and organization. The common thread was that those subjects all require a solid foundation of social thinking. For example, with math problem solving, students might think: "But I got the right answer, why do I need to explain how I got there?" Students need the understanding that the math teacher wants to see that students have the ability to think through

Real examples	Examples of social behavioral challenges	Examples of how it impacts reading comprehension
Jonah, age 8, likes to play kickball at recess, but he gets so caught up with everyone following all the rules that he forgets the goal is to hang out and have fun with friends. The other kids playing understand that concept and enjoy playing together, but Jonah gets so frustrated when a rule is fudged that he does not enjoy the game, and the other kids don't want him to play the next time.	Difficulty speaking coherently and fluidly about a topic; tendency to over-focus on a detail	Difficulty summarizing what was read; getting the "main idea." Discerning the difference between an idea and a detail.
Alex, age 15, wants to fit in, so he repeats off-color jokes in mixed company. He isn't aware that the people are laughing out of discomfort and not because they think he is funny, so he continues to relate the jokes in other settings.	Anxiety, desire to fit in but lack of ability to do so, misunderstanding of interactions, difficulty understanding the difference between fun teasing, mean teasing, and bullying	Difficulty understanding social interactions in stories, how characters interact and why, misunderstanding humor
Dan, age 12, has been having trouble in PE during a basketball unit. Because he is uncoordinated and has trouble getting a basket, much attention is given to him, and it makes him anxious. He reacts by throwing the ball, yelling, and stomping out. During a social group, the students play basketball at the local church. Instead of trying to make the most or best baskets, the group sees who can make the silliest attempt. Anxieties decrease, and Dan enjoys the game and begins to try to make real baskets without the behavioral meltdowns. No special attention is focused on him when he misses, and his confidence improves.		

solving an equation rather than just producing the correct answer. Social thinking is also needed in relation to writing content and organization. When students are given a topic such as "Write a persuasive paragraph to your parents on why you should get more allowance," students with social thinking challenges might answer "so I can get more video games" and "because I don't get enough." An effective answer takes an awareness of the audience, and thinking about what would make mom *want* to give me more allowance. It takes social thinking. With regard to reading comprehension: Reading the words on the page does not indicate that a student can understand the social implications of what happened. Readers need to access background knowledge, connect what they read to themselves and the world around them, understand the characters and the characters' intentions, thoughts, and feelings, and understand the meaning of the social interactions they read about. It is a daunting task. All of these academic tasks require an ability to *think social.*

Social *Skills* versus Social *Thinking*

When my son was diagnosed in 2000, Applied Behavior Analysis (ABA) was the gold standard for intensive intervention for young children with autism. With some guidance from mentors, we found great therapists to help us set up a rigorous home program by the time he was two-and-a-half years old. His progress was remarkable! It was actually because of what I saw ABA could do for a child with autism that I decided to go into the field myself. The idea that you could take any skill, break it down into manageable chunks, teach them to the child with positive reinforcement and repetition, and that child could learn that skill was remarkable. I saw it happen over and over again—how my son would not have a skill that his peers had without effort; but if we taught it to him, he was fully capable of learning and using it. It just had to be taught more systematically.

By the time he was five or six years old, he had a set of core skills from which he could build good social behavior. "Social skills training" was the norm for teaching social behavior at that time. This consisted of the same techniques we used in our home behavior program; that is, taking a skill (in this case, a social skill), breaking it down into smaller parts, and teaching it through repetition and positive reinforcement. We used a lot of puppets and little figurines for this. And it also worked. He gained a set of fairly typical-looking social skills. He was able to navigate many social situations with the tools he had learned.

As he got older, the social expectations grew more complicated, and the nuances of social behavior became subtler. When he was six, he had learned to engage another child by simply asking to play (and the other child would usually agree); at age ten, that whole interaction would depend on *who* he wanted to talk to, *what* that child was already doing, the *history* he had with that child, *when* he should say something, and *how* he presented himself (verbally and nonverbally). It had become much more complex. For example, we had taught him that Saturday mornings he was to sort the clean laundry that was usually in his parent's bedroom. His dad had recently begun working swing shift (usually getting home around 3 a.m.) as a police officer, so on the nights that he worked, he slept in until late morning. On this particular Saturday morning, our son, having learned the behavioral expectation, went into our room early in the morning when he woke up, flipped on the light, and starting doing his chore. He had not thought through what the result of that action would be when his dad was in there sleeping. He had learned the "skill," but the thinking behind the meaning and result of the skill is where he fell short. It became clear to me that simply teaching him *what* to do was not enough. He would have to learn to *think*. In addition to behaving in a socially acceptable manner, he would need to think social.

As I started reading about Social Thinking and going to conferences on the subject presented by Michelle Garcia Winner, I found that her method of teaching Social Thinking addressed my son's and other students' specific needs. She wanted students who had good cognitive skills to go beyond learning social "skills" (as simply behavior) and to learn to actually *think social*. This transformed my whole method of teaching, not only with my son but with all of the students I taught. Basic behavioral principles remained prevalent, especially when working with early learners, but as students gained more social knowledge, expectations, and ability, I began to shift my focus from teaching them not only *what* to do but *why* and *how*.

Because the field of Social Thinking is fairly new, research has been scarce. The research that has begun to emerge supports what I have come to see anecdotally—teaching students to think socially makes a difference in how they act.

In one study (Lee et al., 2009), four teenage males with high-functioning autism were assessed using the Social Thinking-Social Communication Profile™ (ST-SCP) that was developed by Winner's clinic. The researchers used the ST-SCP to evaluate the students using the ILAUGH model. The students were in a group that focused on teaching Social Thinking (following the ILAUGH model) for a total of eight sessions. The students were assessed again at the end of the set of sessions using the same assessment method. While gains were not huge, they were significant in that each student improved across almost all domains in such a short period of time.

In another study (Crooke et al., 2007), which is part of a larger ongoing multiple-baseline treatment study, six pre-adolescent males who had not received prior social skills training took part in a Social Thinking group over eight weeks. This study measured with observable means (outward behavior) the result of the cognitive instruction (inward thinking instruction). Data was collected on verbal and nonverbal social behaviors like on-topic remarks, initiations, and unusual body movements. All subjects showed improvements in expected behaviors and almost all showed a decrease in unexpected behaviors. Some of the improvements were quite significant.

While there are not yet many studies about Social Thinking, the results are promising, and the anecdotal accounts from practitioners, teachers, and parents are overwhelmingly positive. Because this is not a treatment that is learned quickly, real gains take time and evolve. Social learning continues to evolve and should not be seen as a static skill, just as the complexity of reading comprehension also increases with each year of a child's schooling. As Social Thinking becomes more and more the therapy of choice for educators and therapists who work with cognitively-able but socially-challenged students, further research can be expected.

3

Social Thinkers

‖‖‖

Different Kinds of "Thinkers"

It's important to identify what kind of a "social thinker" students are in order to understand them and decide what to teach. For example, students who don't know that eyes show what someone is thinking may be able to be behaviorally taught to make eye contact. However, they will lack the knowledge about *why* it's important and may not *gain information* from that eye contact. As with any teaching, we have to discover where students' learning is, go to that place, and then help—through scaffolding and guiding—move students forward.

Social thinkers come in a variety of shapes and sizes. There are plenty of students for whom a social group setting is not yet appropriate. These are students who may have classic autism, significant impairments, or whose behavior may impede the learning of peers. They may be minimally verbal, and most of their communication relates to their needs and wants and are not communication overtures. These students don't yet show interest in the thoughts or actions of others, are extremely aloof, appear to live "in their own world," and learn most effectively in a structured setting while not gaining much learning from a group environment. These students generally do better in an individual, structured setting working on more concrete prerequisite skills.

It's important to note that diagnoses such as autism spectrum disorders (ASD) and ADHD do not predict a student's social thinking level. Two students who may look identical on standardized tests (cognitive, academic, and language) and share the same diagnosis, may have completely different social thinking. Diagnosis and social thinking are not inextricably connected.

Students who can often be positively affected by social thinking concept instruction can generally be divided into different social thinking categories described in the Social Thinking-Social Communication

21

Profile™ (Winner, Madrigal & Crooke, 2011). Of the six categories described in this scale, individuals at three of these levels are most likely to gain knowledge from specialized reading comprehension teaching strategies: the Emerging Social Communicator (ESC), the Resistant Social Communicator (RSC), and the Weak Interactive Social Communicator (WISC), a subcategory of the Socially Nuanced Social Communicator (SNSC) category. This discussion will focus on two groups: the Emerging Social Communicator (ESC) and the Weak Interactive Social Communicator (WISC). The Resistant Social Communicator (RSC) falls into the range of the high ESC/low WISC; however, these students generally struggle with learning in a group. An RSC will likely need to be taught individually so as to gain more explicit group relationship skills. From the point of reading comprehension, the following strategies can still be helpful as they relate to the RSC as an academic learner.

The Emerging Social Communicator (ESC)

ESC thinkers are usually easily identified as impaired upon first meeting, although there is certainly a range of impairment. On one end of the ESC continuum, they may appear more impaired and aloof but participate and engage more in a highly structured environment. Those on the other end of the continuum may still have an odd affect and appear awkward but can participate in many neurotypical activities and engage appropriately with some guidance. The ESC language is usually delayed; they use literal language and are self-focused in their comments and responses to the world around them. They generally have weak social pragmatic language skills and their speech is overly formal (pedantic). They lack awareness of how they are perceived by others and often have "stranger danger" given their inability to read others' motives and intentions. They also are weak or fail in understanding that people are trying to interpret the intentions of the ESC as well. They don't understand why people form the social thoughts about them that they do.

As far as perspective taking goes, ESCs generally do not have fluid perspective taking skills without explicit instruction. Even when they are taught aspects of perspective taking, they are slow to acquire these concepts and skills and may not find it easy to apply them. Keep in mind that social communication is not merely based on understanding a concept. We have to form and respond to each other within milliseconds; it is an incredibly time anchored concept. Not only do students need to track and monitor what others are thinking and what they know, they also have to be aware of other people's intentions (good and bad). ESCs are inefficient in the perspective taking process. Think of it as trying to solve a social algebraic equation every minute you are around people and how exhausting it would be if you constantly had to do algebra. In social situations, they often misjudge social problems or have a self-centered perception of the problem. These students usually choose to play alone or may join in with explicit instruction, but their processing time is slow. As students get older, typically-developing peers are often unable or unwilling to wait for them to process or react to a social situation. This means ESC students do not have consistent positive social experiences nor do they necessarily understand social expectations.

ESCs struggle to make accurate inferences. They lack the knowledge that others' thoughts are based on different experiences or that people may lie or play tricks on each other. Therefore, they find it difficult to understand what others think or feel and what they might intend to do on a playground, in a classroom, or even at home. It's hard for an ESC to identify another person's emotions and thoughts and then change his or her own behavior to adjust to what they think others might be thinking. They need extensive teaching to begin to understand these concepts and even more to apply them. Their lack of perspective taking ability logically impacts their ability to predict and infer what others are doing or thinking in their presence or what is implied in a textbook. It is not uncommon for an ESC to be diagnosed with hyperlexia, the ability to decode with great fluency while not comprehending well what they are reading.

In a group setting, these students often struggle with what Winner (2005) refers to as keeping their brain and body in the group. They also have difficulties when they play games that involve winning, losing, and being flexible. In general, ESCs can learn many of these skills but often appear awkward in applying them even after extensive training.

Examples of the ESC

Antonio. Antonio is a nine-year-old boy with autism and hyperlexia. He can decode words well above grade level, but his reading comprehension is low. He speaks in simple sentences, often fragments. Although he can answer concrete questions, he has difficulties with answering abstract questions such as *why* and *how*.

23

He greets peers when instructed to do so but generally doesn't do this on his own. When observed in a social setting with a group of peers, Antonio usually plays on his own. He is more than happy to engage when prompted though he doesn't think to do this when left to his own devices. Antonio can be taught to understand and explain what people might be thinking in a specific situation; however, he does not generalize this to other aspects of his day or learning scenarios. Antonio needs adult intervention to help navigate most social problem situations that arise. Antonio benefits from a visual schedule because he cannot predict what will happen next in his school day and needs treatment tools such as social stories to help explain expectations driven by specific situations and the people within them.

James. James is an eight-year-old boy with high-functioning autism. His speech and language development are measured to be at age level, but his communication skills are low as he does not seem to be aware of the need to have back-and-forth conversation with a partner. James perseverates on building structures and traveling and talks incessantly about them even when his talking partner clearly shows a lack of interest. When with a group of peers, James seeks to dominate the play with his perseverations. If peers do not join with him, he is more likely to play by himself than to change any part of his intended play routine. James does not appear to feel bad when his peers do not want to play or interact with him, nor is he aware when his behavior sets him apart from his peers. He has little awareness that the people around him are having weird or uncomfortable thoughts about him.

Shauna. Shauna is a nine-year-old girl with high-functioning autism. Cognitively, she is within the average range but struggles with writing organization, math problem solving, and general organizational skills. Shauna can pass as "normal" at times because of her good language skills, although if you listen closely, you'll hear that most of her language is self-centered and less responsive to a partner than might be the case with a typically-developing peer. Shauna wants to fit in and will engage in inappropriate, attention-seeking behavior to try to engage her peers. She is aware of how other people have thoughts in their heads that are different than her own, and she even understands that her behavior can change the way people think and feel, while struggling with understanding why that is important. Though she knows the "right" answers in a structured, learning setting, she doesn't readily apply those skills in a real-life situation.

The Weak Interactive Social Communicator (WISC)

Once students begin to gain some perspective-thinking skills, they also attain some ability to infer and make predictions. These students can "fake" typical in that they can often pass for typically-developing students with a cursory glance. You often can't pick them out of a crowd unless you really know what to look for. However, their social learning challenges become apparent upon deeper examination, particularly in the area of social interactions. They are usually at or above grade level academically while still struggling with some aspects of reading comprehension, writing organization, language-based math concepts, and executive function tasks like organization and study skills. Many of these students are argumentative given their awareness of their innate academic intelligence. However, they lack insight into the more subtle ways they are expected to blend into a group as the social mind and related expectations grow and expand with each year (if not month) of childhood. These students have more awareness of social information but lack an understanding of what they do (or fail to do) that impacts the perception of others.

WISCs appear to be at greater risk for social anxiety and depression because they are becoming aware of their differences while still finding it difficult to know how to make changes or to even care to make changes. They make excuses or pretend they don't care about others' views of them. They may recognize that their behavior affects the emotions and thoughts of the people around them but still struggle with adjusting their behavior to change how other people think and feel about them. In other words, they aren't able to view themselves accurately from another person's perspective. In addition, these students usually have experienced years of unsuccessful social interactions. These failures snowball, making them less willing to learn or try again and causing continued anxiety.

With peers, WISCs often seek to have friends and be accepted but typically have a small group of accepting friends. They either try to overcompensate for peers' attention with increasingly odd behavior or self-isolate to avoid rejection. They're smart so are pretty good at recognizing challenges in others even if they cannot recognize the same challenge in themselves. They can pick up on a lesson quickly and accurately but have problems "in-the-moment" with translating the lesson to reality. They show some rigidity in social problem solving and are gullible and an easy target for teasing.

There is a range of ability in WISCs, with beginners having more glaringly obvious deficits while higher thinkers are beginning to blend into "normal" behavior. It can be a challenge with the higher-level students to decipher whether a certain behavior is clinically significant or just a personality trait.

Examples of the WISC

David. David is a 12-year-old boy with high-functioning autism. He is highly gifted academically but social interactions with typically-developing boys his age are challenging for him. He has a small group of friends who are all a little quirky and forgiving of odd behavior. He does not have consistent interactions with other students outside of school. His speech is a little stilted and pedantic, and he has some dysfluencies (although not enough to require speech therapy). He sometimes uses non-sequiturs or logical fallacies in his communication that adults find comical; peers are not so forgiving. Unless he has a structured and visual classroom environment, his anxieties increase and make it difficult for him to learn and stay organized. He enjoys school, which he finds easy for the most part though he does not like to be asked to edit his work or be told about his mistakes. He can be argumentative with teachers, not perceiving the different tone of voice he should use with them (as opposed to peers). He tries to gain peers' acceptance by saying something he thinks is funny. When peers laugh because they are uncomfortable or shocked, he perceives it as "liking him." However, when this is pointed out to him, he easily understands, accepts this, and tries to modify his behavior. He learns quickly and easily in a structured setting, but social thinking concepts in real time come a little more slowly.

Samantha. Samantha is an 11-year-old girl diagnosed with PDD-NOS (a form of autism). She has never had a special education plan (an IEP), has never had private therapy, and has "gotten by" so far.

In school, teachers view her as polite and responsible. Samantha has one or two close friends, but without them, she tends to be "on the sidelines" in a social setting. At recess, she usually wanders the perimeter of the playground or engages in a particular play routine with a close friend. Samantha tends to shy away from new social situations by wearing her iPod and "drowning out" the noise and interactions around her. At home, she tends to push her siblings' buttons in a sneaky, subtle way (one of them has autism and tends to melt down easily). She likes to be seen as the "good one" and the rule follower. Samantha wants others to follow the rules and struggles with some inflexibility. Samantha appears fairly happy and well adjusted, but those who know her well understand she is prone to depression and anxiety and would like to fit in better than she does with less effort. For the most part, her differences are subtle and seemingly insignificant. However, it is important to address her difficulties now so she can have the necessary tools as social expectations increase as she gets older.

Michael. Michael is a seven-year-old boy recently diagnosed with Asperger's. He evaded the diagnosis for years because his cognitive abilities were high, and he learned to mask his social ineptitudes by coming across as smart and a little quirky. He learned to read and do math early, though when reading instruction in school began to require more social comprehension, he began to fall behind. He became frustrated and obstinate at school. At recess, at a glance, he appears "typical," generally playing 4-Square with peers. Upon closer examination, it is clear that he tries to control the game and gets mad when it doesn't go his way or he perceives someone is not playing right. However, when he gets "out," he either disputes the call or quits the game. At home, Michael has one or two good friends and gets along well with them. He finds it difficult to make new friends, not really knowing how to engage in small talk and get to know them. He prefers to talk to and interact with adults.

4

Welcome to the Chat Room

||||||||||||||||||||||||||||||||||||||||||||||||||||||||||||||||||||||||||||||||||||||||||||||||||||||||||||||||||||||||||||||||||||||||

The Book Chat

I came up with the Book Chat when I taught special education in elementary school and students came to regularly-scheduled social groups. Because they trickled in before group started, I wanted to get them thinking together in a learning way before starting a social thinking lesson. Picture books with related language-based stories had been helpful to pique the interest of my own son and taught him meaningful skills, so I gave it a try. I would select a book or story to either grab the students' attention or introduce that day's lesson. It became clear that no matter what book I chose, I could incorporate a variety of Social Thinking lessons. I could use a *Captain Underpants* book and the kids would be analyzing the characters and making inferences in no time. They loved it and had no idea how much they were learning from Professor Poopypants.

As a result of this success, I began to include a Book Chat at the start of all my Social Thinking groups, which were held once or twice a week for an hour. It didn't take a lot of preparation. I'd choose a book shortly before group, read through it, and think about what portion to read and what questions I could ask to keep the students engaged and learning. I used my social thinking goals to decide what to focus on and referred to our state educational standards for reading comprehension for guidance on what to teach. We spent about five minutes on Book Chat in the beginner groups and up to twenty minutes in the more advanced groups where we could really dive into a story or concept. The students sat on the floor or at a table in a semi-circle around me. I read the chosen selection to them, frequently asking for their participation but not necessarily having them read any of the text. The focus was on social learning, not decoding, so I did most of the reading. I changed my vocal tones or facial expressions to match the day's goal and to keep students engaged. Book Chats as part of a whole social and academic learning program proved successful, as evidenced by the students' active participation, improvements in their reading comprehension and, most notably, in their increased ability to handle different social situations. When I became a private consultant, I continued beginning social group meetings with a Book Chat, and it continues to be a vital part of all our groups.

Social Thinking Teaching Techniques for the Book Chat

In the years I've been using Book Chats, I've developed a variety of strategies that help me create successful groups and learning targets. The following are some of these techniques.

Social Thinking Vocabulary

Regardless of the lesson being presented or the book being used, Social Thinking vocabulary is woven into everything I do and say in the group. Most of the vocabulary is from the works of Michelle Garcia Winner; however, I frequently introduce new concepts and vocabulary to keep the groups thinking socially. The goal in a Book Chat is to intertwine reading comprehension and social thinking, so I use phrases like, "I like how Justin listened to Jack's comment with his whole body," "Our group was really thinking together to come up with those ideas," and "Oh, I know Brandon is thinking about you when you talk because I can see his eyes looking." Some of the most critical Social Thinking vocabulary terms are explained later in this book.

Choosing Books

The point of the Book Chat is not to improve the students' decoding skills but to teach social thinking through literature and improve reading comprehension (which is usually more delayed than decoding). Select a book that is below the students' cognitive and reading decoding level. Using a book that is easier for students on a cognitive level makes it more likely that they will be able to connect to it and understand it on a deeper level. In addition, a book selection is usually more effective if it includes illustrations that relate to the story.

Look for books that have rich illustrations and characters who are shown to have expressive faces and body language. Some wonderful books in this category are discussed later. I often read less text than is actually written in the book and focus more on artwork, identifying facial expressions, body language, and possible intentions of characters through what students observe in the artwork, text, and my explanations. The artwork depicting characters in most children's literature is exaggerated, which helps the students interpret it.

Using book series that have recurring characters can help students build on previous knowledge. This is typically useful with more capable Social Thinking groups. Often these students find it difficult to connect to characters or situations that differ from their own perseverative interests. Using books whose characters remain constant or ones in which a common theme continues from chapter to chapter can help students with this skill.

Selecting Books for the ESC

When it comes to book choice and reading, ESCs generally like to read a certain genre or style of book if they like to read at all. Because these students lack perspective taking skills, they often choose to engage in books that relate to their obsessive interests or books in one particular genre. They lack the skills to get into the mind of a character, to feel and empathize, to predict what might happen next, to make inferences, and to make connections from one book to another or between their own life and the story.

For the ESC, the Book Chat should focus on creating an enthusiasm for literature, broadening their book choice preferences and interests, and learning to view books as a place to access social learning. Reading comprehension goals may include early inferencing skills, making predictions, accessing previous knowledge, making text connections, and analyzing pictures. Social thinking goals may focus on responding to a partner's request (joint attention), group coordination, looking at characters (in words and pictures) and their body language and what their environment is saying, identifying expected and unexpected behavior, identifying how one's behavior has an effect on others, making smart and wacky guesses, and a beginning understanding of social rules as exemplified in the literature. Examples of good book choices and how to utilize them are included later in this book.

Selecting Books for the WISC

For the student whose symptoms are starting to overlap with typical behavior, the Book Chat literary choices can be more advanced. By this stage in development, the learning challenges are generally complex. It's one thing to teach a student to think about the effect of his behavior in a game of 4-Square at recess and quite another to teach him to understand the social make-up of young teenage girls!

Make sure to include a variety of age-appropriate books. For this group, books that are longer and contain more complex stories work well. These books can span multiple sessions, which will also help the students retain and recall previous learning. Books should have fewer pictures because the students will be learning more from the author's perspective and intent. Reading comprehension goals may include more advanced inferencing skills and making predictions, accessing previous knowledge and applying it over multiple sessions, making text connections, especially if students can connect to their own social lives, and synthesizing and summarizing stories. Social thinking goals may focus more on the social dynamics of peers and observed situations. This group will learn more about how their behavior affects the people around them and how they can modify what they do to keep people thinking about them in the ways they would like. Examples of good book choices for this group can be found later in this book.

Using Declarative Language

Imperative communication is anything that demands a certain response from a communicative partner. Examples are questions ("What are you doing?") and requests ("Please put that down"). Imperative communication does not take a lot of thinking. It just assumes a response. Imperative communication can create anxiety if a student tries to give the "right" answer but is unsure of the answer or the expected response. *Declarative* communication is used to make comments and express feelings and thoughts. Such communication is intended to share experience. For example, "It looks like it's going to rain today" and "I'm really worried about that" are comments that express feelings and thoughts and usually promote conversation with a partner. It requires an ability to infer. Neurotypicals (persons with typical development) use declarative language about 80% of the time and imperative language about 20% of the time. However, children with social cognitive disorders hear and use about 95% imperatives. Think about how we talk to children: "Sit here." "Don't touch that." "What did you do today?" "Go get your brother." In changing what language we use to incorporate more declarative language, we not only help them begin to make inferences and improve perspective taking but also prepare them for the model of typical conversation, which is primarily declarative. Declarative comments might be "I see your friend is sitting here and there's an open spot next to him." "Whoa! I love it when you ask me if you can play with that!" "Today I went to the store and then got a car wash." "I'm ready to have dinner."

The same concepts can apply when doing Book Chats. Imperatives are often necessary, but whenever possible, use declarative language. Comments like "I wonder if...," "That would be really cool if...," "Look! It's a...," and "I see that ..." will provide students with an opportunity to really *think* and develop their own conclusions. Responses are invited but not demanded, so anxiety decreases.

Allowing Time for Processing and Engagement
Along with using declarative language, it's important to give students time to process and think. There is no rush and nothing wrong with a little silence. Pause. Give students time to think. Present a thought, and then let the students chew on it. In addition, if you are losing "brains" in the group, an elongated pause can go a long way to get them orienting back to the group. A long pause is unnatural, and it may cause a daydreaming student to snap back to reality.

Also, stop throughout the story to ask questions and analyze concepts. A short story could take a long time if needed. Don't feel you have to finish a book in a certain amount of time if the students are engaged. I can make *Don't Let the Pigeon Drive the Bus* last 20 minutes. Of course, don't drag something out so long that you've lost the students' interest or engagement in your learning objectives. If you need to stop a book before you finish because you've run out of time, go ahead. You can always come back to it at your next session. This can also help students work on carrying over previous knowledge.

Being Animated

Use animated facial expressions and a high affect as you read. Act excited about the book. How can you expect your students to engage and connect if you're droning on about some character you obviously don't care about? Often when I read a story, I suddenly stop, gasp, pull the book into my chest, and look around at the group with wide eyes: "No way! You won't believe this next part!" Lagging eyes come back to me with interest.

Contributing Ideas

Make sure *all* the students in a group contribute ideas. It's difficult to assess student learning without input. This is a good time to work on the skill of identifying who someone is thinking about by looking at the person's eyes. At times I have students raise their hands to answer, but mostly I teach the students that they know I am asking them a question or am ready to hear their comment when my eyes are directed at them (thinking with eyes). I use a "speak to the hand" nonverbal gesture to other students who chime in when my eyes are focused on another student. This may seem rude to an untrained onlooker, but students with social cognitive disorders need to be taught clearly what is expected. They don't necessarily learn without explicit instruction. It also enables me to continue to direct my focus and attention to the student who I *do* want to talk, so I continue to direct my whole body and face toward that student and not toward the blurter. I also point to the speaker to direct the other students' eyes to that student.

Reinforcing Good Social Thinking

Not every answer has to be correct to show good social and group thinking. Reinforce students when they show they are thinking with the group and being "present," even if their answers may be considered inaccurate. Reward a student's positive participation by pointing out how the contribution makes everyone in the group feel good and how it makes teachers feel positive about their own efforts to teach. I find myself saying things like, "Wow! I hadn't thought of it that way, but you really got me thinking" or "I was thinking of something else, but I really like how you were thinking about the group when you shared your guess!" I use many "I like it when…" statements to show students how it makes me feel good when they have their brains, bodies, and eyes with the group. I make comments like, "Oh, we need to wait just a second so our group can work together to think about this."

Addressing Challenging Behavior

No matter how engaged you keep the students, inevitably some will engage in challenging behaviors. You can't create a mix of students with these difficulties and not have moments of friction. Instead of a long discussion about how to analyze the function of behavior and systematic plans for decreasing behavior, I'll keep it simple: for the most part, often undesirable behaviors can be addressed through one technique—Planned Ignoring. This is the process of ignoring inappropriate behavior while giving additional attention and praise for appropriate behavior. Ignore means not looking, not talking, and moving on.

Planned Ignoring does not mean that the behavior is acceptable, that the rules have changed, or that you are playing favorites by letting someone get away with something. It means that you are in control of determining what is important to pay attention to, and that what you are doing is more important than the undesirable behavior being exhibited.

It's simple. Unless it's a safety issue, if you don't like it, I recommend that you don't talk about it, don't look at it, and don't raise your eyebrows at it. If you do like it, look at it, praise it, and give it attention.

If a disruptive behavior continues, I recommend you use the least intrusive prompt necessary, such as nonverbal cues to correct it. Challenging behavior that requires more intrusive intervention could mean that students aren't quite ready for a Social Thinking group and may need more individualized instruction. This doesn't mean they shouldn't receive Social Thinking instruction, just that they may not be ready to learn in a group setting. *All* interactions are social interactions, and not all students are ready to learn in a larger setting.

Playing with Shared Imagination

Michelle Garcia Winner coined the term "shared imagination" when describing how typically-developing social thinking children play. A "shared" imagination differs from a "singular" imagination in a variety of ways. A singular imagination is self-contained in one's own mind and view of the world. Students can adapt and change it as they choose and see fit. In contrast, a shared imagination involves creating ideas outside of current reality jointly with at least one other person. To do this effectively, one has to have some level of skill in perspective taking. One of my students who has an incredible imagination calls himself "captain" and enacts great, elaborate scenarios of himself on a variety of ships and with grand missions. When left to play with other students, however, he makes little to no effort to involve them in his play. If prompted, he tries to dictate to them what to do and say, not in an effort to have cooperative imagination, but to make them a part of his thought process. This is a singular imagination. A shared imagination comprises a lot of "what ifs" and "what should we do" and joint decision-making. It involves being aware of the partners' thought processes and how they think things are going and what should be done next. It's a collaborative effort that is difficult for students with social cognitive challenges. This concept is especially hard for the ESC students.

To work on this concept (and many others), I often use "thought bubbles" in our social thinking groups. One way I do this is to draw a large thought bubble on paper and put it in front of the students. As we read, we all add what we are thinking about to the group thought bubble. I also use individual thought bubbles to illustrate how each of our thoughts and images may differ somewhat from each other. Beyond that, there are good books that lend to teaching the shared imagination concept. Students describe aloud their reactions to a selection you have read or the group can act it out, encouraging each other and sharing ideas as they do so. When working on this concept, I use a lot of "keeping your brain in the group" language to remind students to think together as a group.

Developing a Sense of Wonder

Students with social cognitive difficulties may develop a sense of wonder when it comes to academic endeavors, especially if they are high academic students. Some refer to this as "science wonder." However, these same students seem to have developed little to no sense of wonder or curiosity when it comes to social interactions. For example, when I bring out the book *Ripley's Believe It or Not!* or *Guinness World Records,* students in my groups are fascinated and ask probing questions about what we read about. They even make some great connections to their own lives ("My uncle grew a squash that was 20 pounds!"). However, if I present any number of social situation picture cards, you can almost hear crickets in the room where previously conversation had buzzed. Students may not understand the social situation to begin with, but beyond that, they have no natural interest to find out more, to develop that sense of curiosity and wonder. It's unnatural for them.

This skill can be targeted through literature as well as with real-life practice. I use thoughtful, leading probes such as, "Gee, I wonder if …," "It's interesting that …," and "Hmmm, I think I would have…." Encourage students to take a chance and make guesses and then to be okay if guesses turn out to be wrong. Positively reinforce any effort to think ahead and to show curiosity. When I first start doing Book Chats with new students and ask them to make a "smart guess" about what a character might do in a situation, the answer is almost always "Turn the page and find out!" They don't know how to brainstorm, analyze, and make guesses and, because of this, they don't learn from their curiosity.

Problem Solving

In real life, students with social cognitive challenges often struggle with the prerequisite skills for personal problem solving. They often don't look at a problem realistically. One common mistake I witness is that students think a problem is much bigger than it is. One student completely melts down if someone even looks like they might be cutting in line: yelling, screaming, crying, pointing fingers. His reaction is so big and out of sync with the size of the problem that he further ostracizes himself with his response. In addition to not understanding the problem, students may not accurately identify cause and effect, may not make correct predictions according to the social situation, and may not make inferences based on subtle nuances. All of this contributes to making it difficult to solve their own social problems.

Children's literature is riddled with social problems. Skilled readers recognize social problems in literature and quickly and efficiently brainstorm possible solutions before the author presents the real solution. When the solution does appear, skilled readers then reanalyze their own hypotheses and decide how appropriate they were. They learn, and the next time they use that knowledge to make even better guesses. Students with social learning challenges may not recognize that a problem situation has been presented and will likely not be able to brainstorm efficiently or effectively about possible solutions. You can give students frequent opportunities to make guesses about possible solutions to problems. In addition, you can help them relate social problems they encounter in literature to their own social problems in real life. I like to use the Social Behavior Map (Winner, 2005) to help students identify, in literature as well as in real life, what a problem situation may be, what would be the expected and unexpected reactions, how it makes them and others feel, and what are the natural consequences of certain choices.

Putting It All Together

The social world comes at us quickly. There is no time in a real-world situation to analyze and come up with an expected social response unless we do it seamlessly. In the adult world, people may be more forgiving of differences in social processing (at least when it comes to children), but kids don't easily forgive or give second chances to each other. It is essential that we teach students who have social cognitive differences to think accurately and to respond automatically. The Book Chat is one tool to use when teaching social thinking in a controlled environment.

The Book Chat presents social situations for students to analyze that are not happening "right now." Doing this provides an opportunity for slower processing. Students can be introduced to a social situation, pause the situation, think about it, talk about it, come up with expected responses, and even practice responding. This can never be done in real time! Just slowing down a social situation may give students a chance to stop and think, which may give them a sense of success and confidence. Many of these students struggle with anxiety and depression that often stem from a history of the inability to respond appropriately in social situations. Slowing it down and giving them a chance to learn at their own pace can be a remarkable confidence booster.

Working on social thinking in a group can be great for peer bonding and forming friendships. Students are "down in the trenches" together, battling their own little social war. Students will find some of the same skills hard to learn, they will make similar mistakes, and some will need the same repetition to acquire a skill. They explore together, learning from one another. For some, this may be their first successful and productive interaction with peers. As they work together, there is a sort of synergy. The group works better and becomes *more* than any combination of the individuals.

The Book Chat is also an opportunity to be the "bomb squad." Potentially difficult and stressful social scenarios can be presented in a controlled environment. These can be worked out and "diffused" in the presence of an educated adult and often peers who are learning the same skills. This is particularly helpful when dealing with situations that cause anxiety or stress for the students. A stress-inducing situation can be introduced through literature, characters dealing with the situation can be observed, and the students can look at the situation from a step back. They have a better chance of looking at the situation more objectively when they're not actually *in* the situation. They learn and practice and talk through their anxieties and stress through the guidance of a skilled facilitator. When a similar situation comes up in real life, they have some tools to help them respond.

5

Educational Standards, Reading Comprehension, and Social Thinking

‖‖

Measuring Success in the Classroom

With today's focus on national and state educational standards, it is appropriate to develop learning targets and teaching methodology that relate to those standards. Setting high standards and creating measurable goals helps us to create targets and measure our success in teaching those targets. The important question to address is, "Are the students learning?"

Today's way of measuring success began with a movement in the 1980s called "outcome-based education," also known more recently as "standards-based education." Previously, the focus had been on what was being taught and the materials and services that were available to students. The new thinking focused on what the students learned, with less emphasis on the method used to get there. In August 1981, the National Commission on Excellence in Education was given the task to investigate the quality of learning and teaching in the nation's schools. Their report, *A Nation at Risk* (U.S. Dept. Ed., 1983), concluded that there had been a decline in the quality and outcome of education standards. Their report recommended changes: the *content* of what is being taught should be strengthened, *expectations* of students' success should increase, the *time* students are expected to be engaged in learning tasks should increase, and the field of *teaching* should be made more stringent and rewarding for qualified teachers. This was the beginning of an evolution in achievement testing and standards-based education.

By 1994, the Improving America's Schools Act of 1994 (IASA) reauthorized the Elementary and Secondary Education Act of 1965

(ESEA), which focused federal funding on low achieving schools. By the late 1990s, almost all states had adopted standards in at least reading and math. With the adoption of No Child Left Behind or NCLB (2002), which required more accountability, local control, parental involvement, and federal funding, all states were required to adopt standards and account for students' progress towards those goals. National standards were not set, but each state was required to adopt their own state standards and demonstrate that state's learning progress. Although there has been a lot of controversy about the implementation of NCLB, what is clear is that the use of educational standards is now *the* "standard" in the public education of the nation's students.

Reading Comprehension Strategies

Many reading comprehension strategies have been adopted in recent years. However, some are more practical when teaching students with social cognitive challenges for targeting their core deficits. Some of these strategies are described next.

Building on Prior Knowledge

This vital strategy helps improve a student's ability to infer. Building on prior knowledge means using one's own past experiences and learning opportunities (schema) to create an understanding of a current situation. From my experience, students with social cognitive difficulties generally live "in the now." They have to be presented with all the information, and they need to have it in front of them to make sense of the big picture. I can read a chapter from a book and have the students engaged and excited, but by the next week's group, they find it challenging when I ask them to recollect that information. They may give scattered responses about details we had discussed or read or may simply give me blank looks as if we've never read it before. Or, when we read a story about a family going to the beach, the students in the group struggle to identify their own experiences with going to a beach. Without those skills, making sense of literature, either fictional or as part of any academic experience, will be greatly hindered.

Building on previous knowledge is being able to retrieve what is stored in one's brain and pull vital information and apply it effectively. This skill takes a long time to develop. I use a strategy called "people files" (Winner, 2005) in my Social Thinking groups to teach that we all have "people files" in our heads in which we store information we know about one another. Then, when we interact with someone, we pull the information we have in that file to know how to better communicate and build a relationship with that person. This concept can be used when doing Book Chats. "Do you remember what is in Henry's friend's file about Josie?" The students have to retrieve what they remember about previous interactions between the characters, what Henry thought of the interaction, and what he placed in his friend file about Josie. They then have to analyze how that information is useful and relevant in this new situation.

Choral Reading and Cloze Activities

Choral reading is group or unison reading aloud. Cloze activities involve reading or listening to a text in which some words are removed and having to figure out what word fills in the blank for the text to make sense. These are both techniques I use mostly when I'm trying to improve initiation of language.

For example, with beginning ESCs, just getting them to participate in a group setting may be the primary goal. This may be their first experience in a group dynamic where they are not just learning to "sit still and be quiet" but are learning to interact and participate during and with a group. For these beginning social thinkers, learning to be aware of the people around them and to coordinate their thoughts and voices with others is a big enough task.

For these beginning social thinkers, I choose books that have repeating lines or a predictable pattern. I begin the reading and emphasize verbally and nonverbally the phrases for the students to say together. Then, as the book goes along, I pause and look expectantly at the students to encourage them to join in. Throughout the story, I pause for longer periods, using nonverbal cues such as holding my hands to gesture that I am requesting something, repeating a line until the students join in, or, as a last resort, stating, "Say it with me…."

As students gain social cognitive competence, cloze activities can be a good way to teach predicting using smart guesses and building on prior knowledge. Providing students with only part of a text and giving them a chance to infer what belongs can help you assess learning. In *Harry Potter and the Goblet of Fire* (2002), when Harry goes into Dumbledore's office and sneaks a peak into the Pensieve (where Dumbledore stores his extra "thoughts"), I tell my students to help me figure out what word is missing in Dumbledore's response to Harry: "_____ is not a sin.... But we should exercise caution with our _____... yes, indeed." From that clue, we can talk about Harry's character traits and what it was that Dumbledore cautioned Harry about.

Generating and Responding to Essential Questions

This technique involves responding to teacher-created questions to help assess students' learning. Generating and answering questions helps clarify, inquire, predict, and also show understanding.

For students who are more advanced social thinkers, the higher-thinking ESCs or WISCs, learning not only to respond to questions asked (of any variety), but to ask questions is an important reading comprehension skill. Many teachers have been taught the KWL technique created by Ogle (1986), originally called "What I KNOW, What I WANT to Know, and What I LEARNED" or "Know, Wonder, Learn." With this technique, students are encouraged to write or express what they already know about a subject or book, think about what they want to know or what they wonder about (very difficult for students with social cognitive difficulties), and then synthesize the information after reading to find out what they learned and if it answered their original questions. This technique provides students with many opportunities to answer and generate thinking questions.

Another strategy called "Say Something" is a form of paired reading (Udvari-Solner & Kluth, 2007). This involves deciding before reading on a certain place in a text where the group will stop and everyone in the group (or pairs of students as described in the book) will contribute "something." This could be a question, a brief summary, a key point, a new idea, or a connection. The text is read, the stopping point is reached, everyone says something, the group discusses it, and then continues on to the next stopping point. Knowing they will have an appointed time to initiate gives students a chance to plan (using executive functioning) what they want to say, and also decreases their anxiety about contributing ideas because it won't be a spontaneous request. Many students battle a tremendous amount of anxiety as part of their nature or as a result of a history of failed social interactions. Teaching them to assert themselves and to take risks is important in healing and learning. In the Chat Room, ideas can be presented about social situations that the students are not directly involved in, giving them a little distance to observe and analyze.

Inferencing

Making inferences means drawing a logical conclusion based on clues. With inferencing, students gather clues through verbal and nonverbal means to gain understanding of a bigger picture, learn the meaning of unknown words, make predictions, and draw conclusions. If they don't recognize the clues or can't synthesize the clues, understanding what it all means is impossible.

Typically-developing students make inferences throughout the day all the time. They make inferences based on other students' physical appearance, on a known history, on people's facial expressions, and on body language. The problem is that students with social cognitive difficulties are not proficient at making these inferences in real time, let alone while reading.

To be adept at making inferences, skilled readers analyze characters' beliefs, personalities, motivations, history, and interactions with other characters. They understand *why* something is happening or why someone is doing something as well as the author's point of view or purpose in writing in a certain way. They come up with their own conclusions, anticipating how the author will end the story. They connect what is happening in the story with their own lives and make logical deductions. Students with social cognitive disorders are not proficient at pulling all this information together from a social cognitive perspective. In addition, they get overwhelmed by the sheer amount of information included in passages as reading assignments become longer and more complex as they get older. And thus the same failure cycle begins that they experience in social interactions: a lack of core skills creates anxiety or a feeling of failure; that feeling makes them less capable of learning the skills needed; they experience increased anxiety and a feeling of failure; and on it goes. Often, by then, you have a student who not only struggles to gain the skills but hates working on it as well.

To this end, students with social cognitive difficulties need to be systematically taught to first recognize the verbal and nonverbal "clues" that they encounter. Next, they have to determine whether those clues are important or not and then have to synthesize those clues to get the big picture. Finally, they must recognize and understand what that big picture means and recognize how their social environment expects them to react in accordance with that information. That's a lot to do if it doesn't come easily.

Students learn to analyze each situation presented in a Book Chat and figure out what information is important but not readily apparent. For example, in a Norman Rockwell painting, students observe a social situation and can label an assortment of details in the picture. However, figuring out the whole story of the meaning of the details provides much more of a challenge.

You can teach students to begin making predictions and inferences based on text and on illustrations. This involves pausing regularly and asking questions such as "What do you think will happen next?" and "Why did they do that?" It may be important to know what color Jimmy's shirt was when he went to school that day but not as important as knowing that he likes Suzy, and he knows that Suzy's favorite color is red, so he's choosing to wear that shirt because he wants her to notice him. And it could well be that none of that information was presented explicitly in the text. We have to teach our students to break the "social code." Good questions to get students thinking socially are, "What do we know about…?," "What do you think might happen if/when…," "Why did he say/do that?," "What makes you think that?," "What is she thinking when the other character does/says that?," "How does that make him feel?," and "What do you think will happen next time…?" Words like *believe, think,* and *wonder* are key words.

In addition, look at the illustrations. Illustrators typically are hired to illustrate children's books because of their ability to tell a story through their artwork. The old adage, "A picture is worth a thousand words" really is true. Point out characters' body language and facial expressions, what they see illustrated in the environment, and what they think they might see on the next page.

Making Connections

Students understand text better by making connections to other reading, their own lives, and their own world using their background knowledge. Making connections is a great technique when teaching students to think social. Skilled readers use their background knowledge (past experiences, past reading, opinions, emotions, etc.) to read and analyze information. They make smart guesses through those connections. Keene and Zimmermann (2007) describe the three text connections with which most current teachers are familiar: text-to-text, text-to-self, and text-to-world. Text-to-text means they read something and it makes them think of something else they have read. For example, reading *Chicky Chicky Chook Chook* (MacLennan, 2007) reminds a student of the rhythmic style of *The Banging Book* (Grossman, 1995). Text-to-self is reading something and thinking of something in the student's own life. For example, a student reads *Scaredy Squirrel* (Watt, 2008) and is able to talk about his or her own scared feelings. Text-to-world is reading about something and thinking about something happening in the world. Reading about an earthquake in *Magic Tree House* (Osborne, 2001) makes a student think about an earthquake that happened last month in Tokyo. Teaching students how to do this can be a long process that takes a lot of guided and independent practice.

In *I Read it, but I Don't Get it* (Tovani, 2000), the author points out how the content areas of academic studies are often separated once students reach middle and high school. Students rush from one class to another, from history to math to English, and rarely do teachers integrate the subjects. Students are inadvertently taught that their learning in different subjects is self-contained. Typically-developing students may innately learn to synthesize their core knowledge, but many struggling students do not know how to make those links. As a result, what they read in a story remains in that story; they don't tie it to their own life or personal learning, which lowers their reading comprehension.

Making connections can also be a great tool when working on interpersonal relations. Students' understanding of the material will increase when they can identify and make connections to times when they have encountered similar situations themselves. An example of this is when I used *Diary of a Wimpy Kid* (Kinney, 2007) with a middle school group, a story in which a big brother teases and torments the protagonist. One of my students who had not shown interest previously said, "Hey! I have a brother who does that." From then on, he was more interactive in the lesson as I continued to help him make connections about how this character was similar to and different from his brother.

Beyond making text connections, understanding the meaning behind the story structure is vital to comprehension. The basics are taught to all students (e.g., characters, setting, problem, resolution), but teaching students to understand more of the *why* helps them improve social thinking. Moreau (2010) developed an effective way to teach students who struggle with the concept of story structure. The Story Grammar Marker® and Braidy the StoryBraid™ are components of a visual representation system that helps students visually tell the story, provides a mechanism for them to organize their thoughts, and presents a way for them to make connections in the story and between stories. These tools also help them understand the story itself and free up working memory so they can do more thinking. In addition, these methods teach students to learn more about the situations in a story and how characters feel, what plans they make and why, and how thoughts and feelings may change as a story progresses. Moreau and colleagues have found these tools helpful not only in reading comprehension but also for understanding real-life social scenarios.

Making Predictions

Making predictions is taking information from a given block of text and being able to make a smart guess as to what might happen next and why. Many students with social cognitive difficulties struggle with reading comprehension tasks because they do not think beyond the words on the page. They are incredibly concrete thinkers. If the answer does not appear in black and white on the page, well, there must not be an answer. One way to work on this is through making predictions. Students analyze what they see in the pictures and think about what they read in the text to predict what might happen next. This also addresses initiation of language because the students have to take a chance with their guess; sometimes they are right and sometimes they are wrong. It's good practice, and it's okay to be wrong! However, guesses should be "smart guesses" and not random thoughts. This takes a synthesis of thinking with eyes, ears, and brain.

In a Book Chat, this can be done by having students look at the illustrations, recognize body language and environmental cues, and listen to what you read and say. For students who do not learn language in a typical fashion, this may include learning about idioms, sarcasm, and other figurative language. With that information, students can begin to make smart guesses as to what might happen next or how the story will end. They may also begin to identify the big picture without its being explicitly shown or told in the story.

Through making predictions and inferences, students show whether they comprehend the underlying situations in a particular situation or story. If they miss important details, their predictions or inferences may be "wacky" as opposed to "smart guesses." With this information, a facilitator can present the material anew with more leading information to help the students grasp the concepts. I like to use a lot of declaratives when I'm guiding students such as "Hmmm, I wonder what he might do if such-and-such" and "Wow, that boy really looks…." I find that using less intrusive language alleviates some of students' anxiety about getting the "right" answer and also means their brains work a little harder to find it.

Sequencing

Sequencing is being able to figure out in what order details were introduced when rethinking a given text. Students with social cognitive difficulties often need extra practice to know how to sequence events. This may come from a lack of ability to see the big picture. I work on this skill by directly looking at sequencing (for example, showing pictures of washing hands or flying a balloon, etc.), but I also work on it in the Chat Room. I read a simple book and then distribute cutout sentences that describe the story in random order. Students have to work together to piece the story back together, putting it in the correct order. This is great for the actual skill of sequencing and also acts as a great coordinating activity for the group.

Summarizing/Synthesizing

Summarizing is being able to succinctly reiterate what a particular text says or teaches, deciding what details are important and sequencing them in the correct order to retell the story. Synthesizing is combining and integrating new information as it is learned.

These are two related strategies. Summarizing involves understanding the big picture of a text and then being able to put it together in a succinct manner. Synthesizing involves much more than that and may even be the most complex of all reading comprehension strategies. To synthesize, readers understand the words and that the words work together to create sentences, and those sentences work together to create paragraphs, and those paragraphs work together to create a big picture. Furthermore, students draw from their background knowledge, previous experience, knowledge base, and personal feelings and emotions to make sense of that big picture. Students then make connections from that big picture to the current schema (pocket of knowledge) and make some sort of personal conclusion—about whether the information was pleasing or not or useful or not and so forth. I'm tired just thinking about it! For students who don't easily acquire any one of those skills, putting them all together in an organized and understandable fashion is a daunting task.

To work on summarizing, you can use guided practice and leading questions to help students learn to identify the main idea and related details. Although this is a common reading comprehension strategy, I find I need to use text far below the students' actual reading level for them to progress. Often, I have to use simple text and even multiple choice answers for students to get the idea. I use text with simple paragraphs without pictures and even picture books with and without text.

Synthesizing is like putting together a puzzle. Usually, you start with the easy pieces, the edges. Once you place them, you work on other pieces that may look alike. When you get big chunks put together, you then try to put them together in the bigger frame. Eventually, you're putting down small, single pieces, but by then you have a good idea of where you are going. Synthesizing is taught through all of our reading comprehension and social thinking instruction. Piece by piece, students learn, and we assess, and we change our teaching according to what we understand the students are learning.

One way you can worked discretely on this ability is by using a book and "speaking your thoughts" as you read. In the beginning of a book, you may have certain inferences or text connections; as you go along in the book, you can verbalize when your thoughts and feelings alter, when your "schema" changes. You modify your thinking as you gain more knowledge and use a variety of strategies to change your schema. After finishing a text, you can then ask the students what they remember your thoughts were in the beginning of the story and how they changed as you came across new information.

Visualizing
Students make mental images regarding what they are reading to comprehend and engage in the text. They adapt and change their mental images as they gain more knowledge. Using eyes and brain is required when students are learning to visualize what they read and hear. Visualizing involves picturing in your mind what is happening in the text. These pictures help the content become real for the students. The pictures should also change as the students gain more information. While many students with social cognitive differences are visual learners, many are less capable of creating their own visualizations if they haven't experienced something similar. For example, a student may be able to picture a cow, but having an image of a pink cow or a cow with wings or a planet of cows would be more difficult. Teaching them to use their eyes and ears to start with information and then to use their brain to add to a mental picture will help them learn this skill.

In my Book Chats, I ask a lot of questions that require students to verbalize their visualizations. I might ask, "So, what do you think so-and-so looks like?" or "If you haven't been to a [place], what do you think it would look like?" I also do mini-visualizing lessons

49

in which I give everyone a piece of paper and have them draw something specific, such as a long snake with spots, then a field of bubbles around the snake, then a miniature person doing something silly to the snake. I try to push the students to do something fun and zany to give them a chance to visualize something outside their own comfort zones. When we're done drawing, we all take turns sharing and observe how everyone's pictures are a little different but they all followed the directions. It's a fun activity!

6

Body in the Group

This chapter and many of those that follow introduce an assortment of tools, techniques, and literature examples to help you establish a Book Chat in almost any Social Thinking, reading comprehension, counseling, or speech therapy group for students with social learning differences. Each chapter begins with a brief summary of a core Social Thinking vocabulary component to target (Winner, 2005). This definition is followed by specific examples of books and reading comprehension strategies you can use in a Book Chat to address that area of Social Thinking. For more detailed information about Social Thinking vocabulary, refer to Winner's publications listed in the References chapter.

The example books and suggested strategies are not intended to be an exhaustive list—there are so many books from which to choose and a multitude of different ways to use them to teach social thinking and reading comprehension. Many books can function to target any one of many goals and can be used with a variety of the strategies. In fact, most books can be used to work with students on a number of skills, and many components of social thinking also overlap. Specific goals that combine reading comprehension and social thinking can be found in Chapter 22: Reading Comprehension and Social Thinking Goals.

Definition
Keeping your body in the group means you are physically present in the group in a way that people *think* you are physically part of the group. Turning your back on a partner or having your body so far away that people don't think you are part of the group can make people have weird or uncomfortable thoughts about you. Keeping your body oriented toward the group or a speaking partner gives them the feeling that you think who they are and what they are saying is important and makes them more likely to engage with you again in the future.

Book Examples

Howard B. Wigglebottom Learns to Listen
by Howard Binkow, Susan F. Cornelison (illustrator)

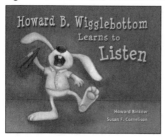

For young and early social thinkers, Howard B. Wigglebottom is a good example of body not in the group. Howard bounces instead of listening during story time, doesn't heed good advice from teachers and friends, and in the end, gets in trouble and is put in time-out. Howard decides he doesn't like being alone and in trouble, so he makes up his mind to do better the next day (which he does).

This story is simple, straightforward, and great to use with early social thinkers. This is also a good book to use to talk about "Energy Hare-y" (see Chapter 18: Superflex and the Unthinkables).

Questions to ask. What are Howard's friends thinking about him when his body is out of the group? What do their faces tell you? How is the teacher feeling? When his friend tries to talk to him, what do you think the friend feels when Howard doesn't listen? What do you think the friend will do the next time the friend wants to talk? What happened to Howard's friend during painting time? How did Howard change his behavior? How do you think that changed the way people were thinking about him?

Personal Space Camp
by Julia Cook, Carrie Hartman (illustrator)

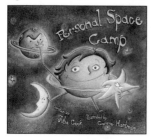

While many of the books I use are not written to address the specific topics we cover in group, this book is a valuable lesson on body space. It is a good choice for an elementary-school age high ESC or WISC group. These should be students who are aware of their body and how it can affect others but may not recognize their own space difficulties. The story is about a boy named Louis who lacks an awareness of personal space and non-maliciously bumps into peers, upsetting both them and the teacher. The teacher sends Louis to "personal space camp" with some other students where the principal teaches them about personal space through the use of visuals like hula hoops and ropes. Some great insights are shared. For example, the principal blows some bubbles and asks if they are all the same size. She explains that one's comfort bubble will not always be the same size—sometimes it will be big, like around a new person or in a new situation; at other times it will be smaller, like around family or friends. The principal also has the students cut out their body shapes from butcher paper and then lays them all out on the circle-time carpet. She points out how hard it is to fit everyone's body on the carpet when they're prostrate like that and says that's why it is important to keep your body space when sitting together with friends on the carpet. The book has excellent illustrations and insights to share.

Questions to ask. What are Louis's friends thinking when he bumps into them? Does Louis notice the expressions on his friends' faces and what they are showing with their body talk? Was personal space camp what Louis thought it would be? How did he react to the unexpected situation? How do you think Louis will change his way of thinking? How will it change his friends', teacher's, and mom's feelings and thoughts about him?

7

Boring Moments

Definition

We all have to do things or participate in activities that we don't find stimulating. There are just some boring things we all have to do. This is an important concept for students to learn because many things they are asked to do are not on their own personal lists of priorities. Sitting in a group in school generates a lot of boring moments, but it doesn't mean students are allowed to announce they are bored or get up and leave an activity. To enable a teacher to teach many different brains the same lesson, there is an unspoken agreement that students will learn to make the best of the "boring moments."

Book Examples
I'm Bored!
by Christine Schneider, Hervé Pinel (illustrator)

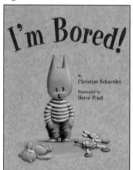

Targeted to the young and early social thinker, *I'm Bored!* offers a concrete example of what to do when you're bored. Little Charlie has a boring Sunday to deal with, and his mom and dad are not helping. When some of his toys become animated and begin complaining that all he does is grumble about being bored, Charlie gets creative and uses his imagination to conquer boredom. His mom is not entirely happy with the mess he creates, but boredom is defeated!

When you introduce the concept of boring moments to students, you can use this book to illustrate what students can do during "down" time. I talk about some of my boring moments. "Oh! Doing the dishes is so BORING! I need your help to figure out how to be like Charlie." I then have the students help me think of fun ways to do the dishes, the laundry, and the grocery shopping. I've heard great responses like, "See how big of a bubble you can make with the dish soap" and "Count the number of items you put in your grocery cart" (from a numbers person, of course). Because students seem to understand this particular type of boredom (e.g., nothing to do), you can use this story as a segue into talking about socially boring moments. Sometimes we find ourselves in situations that bore our brains! Maybe someone is talking about something that doesn't interest us or we have to listen to a teacher talking about a subject we don't like.

Questions to ask. How did Charlie use his imagination? How did it help him? How can this help us learn how to be good social thinkers when we have boring moments? Why is it important to show interest in something in which we're not really interested?

Beatrice Doesn't Want To
by Laura Numeroff, Lynn Munsinger (illustrator)

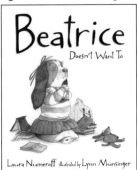

This book is good for the early elementary-school age higher-social thinking students. Henry has to take his younger sister to the library while he does homework. But the library is so boring! Beatrice complains ("I don't want to!") and bothers Henry incessantly. Finally, he has an idea. He takes her to story time where Beatrice, although initially bored, learns to listen to and laugh at the story. By the end, she doesn't even want to go home.

This story focuses on the boring moments we experience daily and how we can do things we don't really want to do in a socially appropriate manner. Henry's and Beatrice's body language are expressive and provide great examples of varying emotional states. I ask the students to notice what Beatrice is expressing with her body language and what the other characters are communicating nonverbally.

Questions to ask. Why do you think Beatrice doesn't like going to the library? What does Beatrice's body say? Why is Beatrice so close to Henry's face? What is Beatrice making Henry think? What are the other kids thinking when Beatrice is standing in the middle of the room? How and why do Beatrice's feelings about the library change? How will the next trip with Henry be different?

8

Expected/Unexpected Behavior

||||||||||||||||||||||||||||||||||||||||||||||||||||||||||||||||||||||||||||||||||||||||||||||||||||||||||||||||||||||||||||||||||||||

Definition

Although this concept is often referred to as "acceptable" and "unacceptable" or "appropriate" and "inappropriate," the terms "expected" and "unexpected" are preferable because they don't elicit an emotional judgment. Each situation has a set of hidden rules that dictate what is expected for each of us to do in that environment to keep people having good thoughts about us. Expected behavior is just that— what society expects from a contributing member of society in a given situation. Unexpected behavior can get us into trouble or give people uncomfortable thoughts about us, making us less able to negotiate society's expectations. Each classroom is a society. Each family is a small society. We behave in such a way as to keep people thinking about us in the way we want them to think about us.

Book Examples
No, David!
by David Shannon

Typically used with the youngest or the early social thinker, this is a simple book that illustrates unexpected behaviors and can be a means to identify how behavior affects the emotional state of others. David is a mischievous little boy who constantly gets into trouble. Throughout the book, his mom tells him "No" and "Come here this instant." In the end, his mom wraps him in a loving embrace because she does love him despite all his naughty antics.

No, David! has terrific illustrations that depict unexpected behaviors such as climbing to get a cookie jar and tracking mud into the house. Because the unexpected behaviors portrayed are obvious, this is a great way to introduce the concept of expected and unexpected behaviors. The book offers many opportunities to analyze illustrations—what they mean, why the behaviors shown are considered unexpected, and what might be their result. I use expressive facial features and clear voice tones when reading to exemplify what the mom is *feeling*. For a somewhat higher-level group, I do a comparison by reading some text without feeling, in a monotone voice, and then reading the same text with high affect and facial expressions that fit the feeling. In the end, I talk about how David's behavior affected how his mom felt at the time, but it never made her stop loving him. Some students with social cognitive difficulties, especially the higher social thinkers, battle depression and low self-esteem because they become aware of how different they are. It's important to reinforce that they have self-worth no matter how difficult it is for them to become a social thinker. There are several other *David* books, all equally engaging.

Questions to ask. What could happen if David climbs up there to get the cookie jar? What could he have done before he came in the house with mud all over? Why is his mom upset about the water on the floor? What might happen if he plays ball in the house? What did happen? How is David feeling now? Why?

Hunter's Best Friend at School
by Laura Malone Elliott, Lynn Munsinger (illustrator)

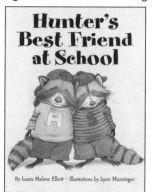

In this story, Hunter's best friend Stripe starts making some poor choices at school, seeking attention in all the wrong ways. The protagonist Hunter joins in a little and decides it's not for him. Hunter's mom suggests that he be a good example for his friend, and maybe Stripe's behavior will change (it does).

In the beginning of this story, the two friends are shown hanging out together, doing the same things, and enjoying each other. In the first two-page spread, Stripe begins to engage in unexpected behavior during circle time. This is the first time you see Hunter's body language and facial expression express frustration. However, Hunter finds himself pulled into the unexpected behavior. Hunter is torn. He wants to fit in with his friend, but he doesn't feel good when he behaves that way. The book shows evocative facial expressions and body language as Hunter goes through this process. The book offers many opportunities to talk about how the other characters are feeling and what they are thinking as a result of Hunter's and Stripe's actions. In the end, Hunter makes good choices and becomes an example and a positive influence on his friend. This is an excellent choice for early elementary-school students. You can simplify it for the mid-ESC or make it more complicated, incorporating more inferencing for the higher ESC or WISC.

Questions to ask. Does Luna look like she's having fun when she's being chased in the beginning? Why didn't she want to be chased later? What is Hunter's body saying after he tears up his frog? What does the teacher think? What is his mom thinking when she sees Hunter come home sad? How did Hunter influence Stripe's behavior? Why did Luna like being chased at the end of the story?

The Terrible Underpants
by Kaz Cooke

Poor Wanda-Linda! She doesn't have any clean underwear today, so she has to wear The Terrible Underpants (an old, worn-out pair). Her parents assure her that no one will see the terrible underpants, but Wanda-Linda isn't so sure. Of course, it wouldn't be a good story unless that did happen. Through various situations, different people get a glimpse of the underpants, culminating in them being shown on the news so the whole world can see. Wanda-Linda has her own, unique solution to the embarrassment.

This book is good to use with older elementary-school students for discussing thought bubbles and people's reactions to Wanda-Linda's situation. You can also use it to talk about making impressions as well as how what we do and say and how we look have an impact on what other people think and feel when they are around us. This is also an incredibly funny book, and kids love it. It provides many opportunities to make inferences based on illustrations, body language, and facial expressions.

Questions to ask. Why is Wanda-Linda worried about what she's going to wear? Why is it important to her to have nice underpants? What does she think might happen? What kinds of thoughts do people have about her when they do see the underpants? Was her solution to the problem reasonable?

How Rude! handbooks
by Alex J. Packer, Ph.D. and
What To Do guides for kids
by Dawn Huebner, Ph.D., Bonnie Matthews (illustrator)

These books are helpful for building social lessons with older students, typically middle or early high school students with high social thinking.

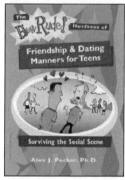

The *How Rude!* books are written for typically-developing teens, teaching them basic manners and social skills (of course, many typical teens could use some manners lessons). *The How Rude! Handbook of Friendship & Dating Manners for Teens* contains some content that would be inappropriate for younger students, and you should always check with parents before delving into topics such as dating and sex (and any other sensitive topics). In addition, it's important to preface these lessons with a discussion about balance. These books are good for introducing positive social expectations, but if taken too literally or rigidly, students may come across as stiff and rule-mongers. No typical peer is fond of a self-appointed social policeman.

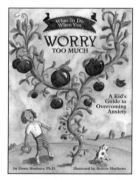

The *What To Do* guides are workbooks for students to use that address such topics as Obsessive Compulsive Disorder and Anxiety. The author uses cognitive-behavioral techniques to help students learn about their own challenges and how to address them. These books are appropriate for almost any age as long as the student is cognitively aware of his or her deficits and is ready to work on them. The books go hand-in-hand with Social Thinking lessons about giving other people good versus weird or uncomfortable thoughts.

The Social Skills Picture Book for High School and Beyond
by Jed Baker and
The Social Success Workbook for Teens
by Barbara Cooper and Nancy Widdows

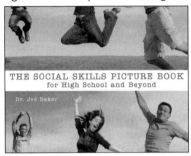

The Social Skills Picture Book for High School and Beyond can be used with students as young as ten. The book present social situations, such as "Knowing When to Stop Talking," followed by three bullet points about the rules that apply; for example, if someone looks bored, ask if he or she wants to hear more. Each rule is illustrated with photos of teens engaged in that social behavior along with thought and dialogue bubbles that address the rule and outcomes. These illustrations show the right way and the wrong ways, or the expected and unexpected ways. In my early teen group, we read and talk about one situation or rule. Some of the students then act out each way and the rest of us guess if they did it the expected or unexpected way.

The Social Success Workbook for Teens by Barbara Cooper and Nancy Widdows is an activity book that deals with such topics as Shades of Anger, When Plans Change, and Developing a Filter (a particularly good one). Each lesson includes a short introduction and workbook activities. There is also a workbook for Anxiety that is helpful.

9

Flexible Brain

||||||||||||||||||||||||||||||||||||||||||||||||||||||||||||||||||||||||||||||||||||||||||||||||||||||||||||||||||||||||||||||||

Definition

Having a flexible brain or "going with the flow" means that you are willing to accept and anticipate change and to create alternative choices for yourself when the world does not work out the way you thought it would. The opposite of a "flexible brain" is a "rock brain" (see Chapter 18: Superflex and the Unthinkables). Michelle Garcia Winner has a saying that "flexible thinking is Social Thinking."

Book Examples

The Odd Egg
by Emily Gravett

In this entertaining book, the animal characters are all laying eggs and getting ready for them to hatch. Duck didn't lay an egg, but she found one. It wasn't an ordinary egg, but she was preparing for it to hatch. However, her friends mock and laugh at her and her funny egg. One by one, the other eggs hatch, and the animals are thrilled with their new arrivals. Soon, Duck's egg begins to crack, and to everyone's surprise, CREAK-CRACK-SNAP! Not a bird, but an alligator emerges and scares all the mocking friends. The end.

Although this book can be used with younger students, it also works with higher-elementary and more adept social thinking students because it is really a metaphorical lesson on flexible thinking. You can ask prediction questions throughout the book, culminating in the arrival of the alligator (always met with a lot of laughs).

Questions to ask. How can you tell the animals are excited about their eggs? Where do you think Duck found her egg? What about the real "owner" of the egg? What do you think happened? Why is Duck thinking about the #1 World's Best Egg prize? Why are the animal friends laughing at Duck? How does that make Duck feel? What is Duck thinking when the other animals' eggs are hatching? When Duck's egg hatches, is it what they expected? What had Duck expected? How did she react?

More Parts
by Tedd Arnold

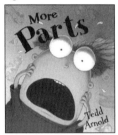

This book offers a whimsical way to learn a variety of idioms and figurative language that are prevalent in the English language. The poor protagonist thinks that his heart is really going to break when he's sad and that he must amputate his hand when asked to "give a hand." He also has to "hold his tongue" and "scream his lungs out."

With beginning social thinkers, I use this book to introduce idioms. We try to make a list of all the idioms we can think of (there are a lot). Higher social thinking students can often identify a large number of idioms and what they mean, but this is a great way to introduce figurative language in general. You can discuss how sometimes people say things that they don't mean or use different tones of voice to mean different things. Students can make connections between their own feelings when they don't understand something to what the boy in the story feels when he doesn't understand the idioms he hears. And, of course, the story elicits many giggles and much group interaction.

Questions to ask. Why was he so confused? How do you think he was feeling as he thought about more and more of his body parts being used in bizarre ways? Have you ever felt confused by something everybody else seems to understand? What are some strategies to overcome the confusion (good segue into being a Social Detective)?

Uncle Shelby's ABZ Book
by Shel Silverstein

This book was originally intended for adults, which is obvious when you read it. You have to be careful in choosing appropriate groups for this book, but it can be a great tool if you choose correctly. It is full of irreverent humor and all sorts of acts one *shouldn't* do, addressed directly to the reader. For example, "A" is for little green apples. "How many nice green apples can *you* eat?" Why is that funny?

One page has a coupon: "Kids! Clip out this certificate and bring it to your friendly neighborhood grocer and he will give you absolutely free . . . A REAL LIVE PONY!" Obviously this is not a book to read to small children, but it can be hilarious for teens and young adults who are developing a sense of humor and are beginning to understand irony. A flexible brain is needed to appreciate Silverstein's wit.

Questions to ask. "How many nice green apples can *you* eat?" What if a friend in your inner circle asked you this question? What would be his/her intent? What if it was someone you've had problems with? What might his/her intent be then? Why is that different?

Diary of a Wimpy Kid
by Jeff Kinney

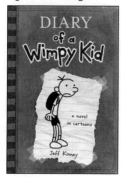

Many students with social cognitive difficulties resist reading any chapter book unless it is about their specific interests or in their favorite genre. However, they are quite willing to read comic books and cartoons. This book, like the others in this series, is a regular chapter book, but the type looks like handwriting, and it filled with line-drawn comic strips that accompany the stories. Because of this, reluctant readers are more likely to engage in the reading and discussion of this story. This book is great for a late elementary or middle school age group. You can use it begin to work on concepts such as analyzing characters, making connections, carrying over story lines, and engaging in a story. The line drawings are quite entertaining and offer much to discuss.

The main character's exploits provide many opportunities to discuss the flexible brain. Greg is new to middle school and trying to find his place in the universe. He is on a quest for status but finds himself thwarted on every side by overbearing parents, an older brother who torments him, a younger brother who annoys him, and nerdy friends. He is small for his age, so his foray into middle school is met by a variety of challenges.

Greg frequently needs a flexible brain; for example, his older brother gets him up for school in the middle of the night, his parents make him take his little brother trick-or-treating, and he is required to wrestle a girl on the wrestling team. Day in and day out, Greg deals with typical middle school challenges that give students in the group a chance to observe and discuss.

Questions to ask. Why is Greg trying to "be cool"? Why is that important to him? How is he learning what to do to fit in better? When does it work and when does it not work? What does he do in each situation?

10

Good and Uncomfortable Thoughts

||||||||||||||||||||||||||||||||||||||||||||||||||||||||||||||||||||||||||||||||||||||||||||||||||||||||||||||||||||||||||||||||||||||||||||

Definition

Throughout the day, we constantly have thoughts about the people around us, and they have thoughts about us. We categorize these thoughts into "good thoughts" and "uncomfortable thoughts." The most important concept here to teach is that we all have the power to change what other people are thinking about us through our behavior to keep them thinking about us the way we want them to. We teach students to notice their own thoughts about others, including us as their parents and teachers. By recognizing we have different types of thoughts, we monitor our own behavior to help people have as good thoughts about us as possible in most situations. However, we all produce some behaviors that create uncomfortable thoughts, often by accident (see Chapter 13: Rubber Chicken Moments).

Book Examples

Come Down Now, Flying Cow!
by Timothy Roland

Typically used with younger students or students for whom inferencing is a new skill, this story helps to work on identifying emotions based on facial expressions and to begin to identify how behavior affects the emotional state of others. Beth the cow is an adventurous bovine. She discovers a hot air balloon, and much to the chagrin of the farmer, she's off on a quest. Despite many mishaps, Beth has a lovely time, although the same can't be said of her traveling pals. Her poor bird friend is worried sick the whole time.

With this book, you can read about and discuss emotions, uncomfortable thoughts, the effects of behavior (expected and unexpected behavior), and making beginning inferences. A variety of emotions are displayed in the story through characters' facial expressions, including surprised, excited, happy, angry, and, especially, worried. In addition to helping the students *identify* the emotions they see, this book can be used to help them to understand *why* the people feel that way. Beth certainly doesn't mean any harm through her adventure, but as a result of her actions, the other characters' emotional paths are changed.

Questions to ask. What is the bird worried about when she points at the kite/the other hot air balloon/the plane? What might happen? Why is the kite boy sad? Where is the fish going to go? How will they help the lady who fell out of the plane? What is the laundry lady saying with her body (before the balloon hits the clothesline)? What is Beth thinking about when she sees the car at the end?

Many of the classic Dr. Seuss books and the Random House Beginner Books® (which look like Dr. Seuss books) are similarly effective for teaching early inference skills. The Winnie the Pooh early books like the Thinking Spot Series (Advance Publishers) and Winnie the Pooh First Readers (Disney Press) have wonderful illustrations of characters who have expressive body language and facial expressions. These books have little text and are great to address reading body language, inferencing, predicting, and identifying good versus uncomfortable thoughts.

Just Me and My Mom
by Mercer Mayer

For the young to middle elementary school student, Mercer Mayer's Little Critter stories are wonderful ways to work on good versus uncomfortable thoughts. In this story, Little Critter is a mischievous anthropomorphic creature reminiscent of Dennis the Menace. He doesn't *mean* to get in trouble, but trouble sure finds him. In this outing with his mom, he loses train tickets, gets kicked out of the museum, brings his frog to a restaurant, and finally falls asleep on the way home, cuddled up to his mom who has been so patient with him.

Mercer Mayer is the master of meaningful illustrations. In all of his books, each page presents plenty to discuss. Throughout the book, you can point out body language, facial expressions, and what is happening in the environment. Most of Mayer's books include recurring illustrations of a spider and/or a frog. Students *love* to locate these on each page. In addition, you can help the students make text connections by asking them what they would do in the situation or what their mom would do if they did what Little Critter did. You can bring in good versus uncomfortable thoughts by asking pointed questions about how the mom might be feeling and what she might be thinking when Little Critter does this or that. The group can talk about the difference between *intent* and *action*. While Little Critter didn't mean any harm, some of his actions cause people extra work or worry or just give them uncomfortable thoughts about him. Students can brainstorm what Little Critter could do differently the next time he goes on an outing with his mom. How would a change in his behavior change the situations he was in?

Questions to ask. What is he or she thinking? What kinds of thoughts are they having about Little Critter? Why? What might happen if he…? Why doesn't his mom want Little Critter to buy the train tickets home? Why is Little Critter tired? How does his mom feel about Little Critter at the beginning of the story? At the end? Why did that change—or remain unchanged?

Any of Mercer Mayer's books can be used in Book Chats with similar goals. Some of the most useful ones are *Just Me and My Dad, I Was So Mad, Just Grandma and Me,* and *Just My Friend and Me.*

11

Keeping Brain in the Group

Definition

Keeping your brain in the group means we can tell you are thinking about what we are thinking about. We notice when people's brains are in the group if their eyes are oriented towards the group or the speaker, their comments are on topic, and they show interest in what the group is talking about or doing. If someone appears to not be listening or looks "spaced out," we don't think that person is thinking with the group and that may give us uncomfortable thoughts.

Book Examples

Go Away, Big Green Monster!
by Ed Emberley

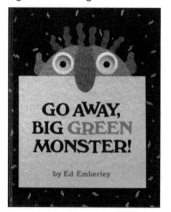

This is an early learner book, good for preschool-age students who are beginning social thinkers. In the first half, the big green monster is created through die cuts, from big yellow eyes to scary teeth. But, don't be scared. The monster is then disassembled through the same process with the repeating phrase, "Go away..."

Early in the book, I simply try to engage students by having them point out their own eyes, teeth, etc. as the monster is created. At the turning point ("You don't scare me!"), I begin emphasizing the text by using a high facial affect and enunciating the "Go away" repeating phrase. Initially, I use a short pause and expectant look to try to get the students to say "Go away" with me. As I go along, I increase my level of anticipation to encourage the students to participate. I lengthen my pauses or draw in my breath and wait before I begin the phrase. If students still don't participate, I reread the same page, requesting a greater response.

The goal is to have the students repeating as a group, which requires an ability to coordinate with a group. If one student says the phrase quickly and another slowly, the group dynamic is lost. Students should not only try to coordinate with you, as the teacher, but also with their neighbors. Sometimes, this can be accomplished by pointing out whose "group voice" was lost and trying the phrase again, really emphasizing saying it together. This helps the students who are just learning to be aware of the impact of people in a social setting. They have to pay attention to more than just the student-teacher relationship but understand that they are one part of a group whole, and they have to work together to succeed.

Similar activities can be done with *Chicka Chicka Boom Boom* by Bill Martin Jr. and John Archambault, *Boom Chicka Rock* by John Archambault and Suzanne Chitwood, and *Are You My Mother?* by P.D. Eastman. These stories work well because they begin with a cloze phrase, and the students can fill in the last word of the repeating phrase as the story progresses. You can expect more and more of the phrase to be repeated together throughout the book. For example, early in *Are You My Mother?*, when the repeating phrase begins, you could say, "Are you my..." and then pause, with the expectation that the students will say "mother" with you. By the end of the book, you may only need to look expectantly at the students, and they should, as a group, repeat the phrase together.

These books are good for helping students to participate and initiate language in a group setting. The predictable pattern in each book will alleviate some anxiety for students who are hesitant to contribute. Speaking out along with the rest of the group gives them a sense of group and causes them to be aware of the people around them.

Mr. Daydream and *Little Miss Chatterbox*
both by Roger Hargreaves

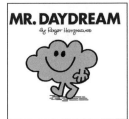

I use these books even with older elementary students, at least those at a high ESC social thinking level. There is a whole series of these small books with clever characters who exemplify everything from curiosity, to being wise, to being helpful. In *Mr. Daydream*, Jack is a little boy who tends to daydream. In school, he lets his mind

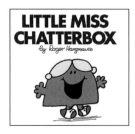

wander, and he meets Mr. Daydream who takes him on a bunch of adventures around the world. He is brought back to reality when his teacher taps his shoulder. In *Little Miss Chatterbox*, a character talks and talks and talks all day long. She gets a job and loses it because she can't stop talking. She gets another, and she loses it. That happens every day for a week. Then, she finds the perfect job—being the "time telling operator" on the phone.

Whether students succumb to daydreaming or to self-centered interests, their brains are out of the group. I like to use these short books to introduce the lesson of "brains in the group." I make up small slips of paper with little brains on them. One of the brains has an X through it. I pass them out privately so students don't know who gets the crossed-out brain. I tell them the person who has the X is supposed to act like his or her brain is out of the group, and we are supposed to try to figure out who it is. We then go on to read a book or play a game, and the students have to keep their guess in their head until I give them the okay. This can be hard. Some of the students who do *not* have the X have a hard time keeping their own brains in the group. And then if some students figure out who has the X, it can be hard for those students to keep the guess in their own head *and* their brain still in the group until the game is over.

Questions to ask. What are Jack's classmates and teacher thinking about him when he's daydreaming? What can he do to change the way they might think about him to get them to think about him in the way he wants? How will that change how he feels about himself?

12

People Files

IIIIIIIIIIIIIIIIIIIIIIIIIIIIIIIIIIIIIIIIIIIIIIIIIIIIIIIIIIIIIIIIIIIIIIIIIIIIIIIIIIIIIIIIIIIIIIIIIIIIIIIIIIIIIIIIIIII

Definition

In our brains, we keep virtual file folders of all the people we know. These files have information about these people—what we know they like, don't like, the type of person each one is. When we have an interaction with one of them, we pull that "file" out of our brain, and we can adjust how we interact with that person based on the information we have about him or her.

Book Examples

Tico and the Golden Wings
by Leo Lionni

With this book, students (typically mid-elementary age) can identify their own talents and struggles and share them in a group setting to build understanding of group dynamics and bond with their peers. In the story, Tico is a bird without wings who wishes for a pair of golden wings. When his wish is granted, his friends mock him and won't talk to him, so Tico goes out on his own. In his travels, he finds someone in need and shares one of his golden feathers. Each time he does this, a black feather grows in its place. When he returns home with wings of black, his friends are relieved to see him. Although he now fits in better, he knows inside there is more to him than the color of his wings.

While similar to *Rainbow Fish* by Marcus Pfister, one way this book differs is that the main character conforms to some extent on the outside while still retaining who he is. You can use it to illustrate that it's important to retain your individuality and unique characteristics at the same time that you are learning to use socially acceptable behavior.

You can read this book and do this related activity with students at the beginning of a social group series. Before reading the book, I prepare a cut-out of a bird with wings whose feathers can be cut apart and put them on different colored paper (each bird on a different color). After reading and discussing the book, I give each student a bird. On each feather, they write something about themselves—something they are good at, something they struggle with, or just something in which they are interested. I monitor the activity to make sure they include a variety of information about themselves. When they are done, they "share" their feathers with their group friends. I show them how to do this by taking one of the feathers and giving it to a student and saying, "Can I share my fear of fast traffic with you?" or "You can have my love of reading." They then share their difficulties, talents, and interests with each other. When sharing is done, they glue their new feathers onto their bird. We take time to discuss how, while we are all unique, we have many things in common, and we can learn and grow together.

Questions to ask. How did Tico feel about himself in the beginning? In the middle? In the end? How and why did that change? Why was it important for him to fit in? What did he learn in the end?

Harry Potter and the Sorcerer's Stone
by J.K. Rowling

For students who are somewhat older and have higher social thinking abilities, typically middle school or older, delving into well-known stories like Harry Potter can be effective. At this level, literature has great social interactions and character developments to explore. If you choose a book like one of those in the Harry Potter series, the content is also interesting.

I don't expect my groups to read a whole Harry Potter book and then work on analyzing it. What *is* fun to do is to get permission from parents to watch the movie. Typically I will stop throughout the movie to talk about what's going on and the characters' relationships. Since most of the students have already seen the movie, we are able to dive deeper into who the characters are and how they think and feel about each other. For a few group sessions following the movie, we have lessons in which we read and use scenes out of the book. Because they have seen the movie, the students are able to retrieve background information to make sense of the reading.

Questions to ask. In *Sorcerer's Stone*, during a scene in the beginning of the book, Harry meets Malfoy for the first time. The movie is visual, and the students can have that scene in their head as I read that part of the book to them. The encounter in the book is much more detailed than in the movie, and I am able to ask targeted questions that help them with the lesson. Where does the scene in the book take place? Why is that different? What do Harry and Ron have in their friend files about Malfoy when they first meet him? What does Malfoy have in his? How and why does this change?

13

Rubber Chicken Moments

‖‖

Definition

Everybody makes small social mistakes. The "rubber chicken" is a visual way to help students realize that it's not the end of the world to make these blunders. You can purchase a rubber chicken at a number of novelty stores and then keep it at the table during group to be used as needed. When you make a blunder, you get to bop yourself in the head with the rubber chicken. Students are not allowed to "hit" anyone else with the rubber chicken, and they are not allowed to intentionally make mistakes so they get a chance to use it. When used appropriately, kids love it and think it's hilarious.

Book Examples

The Recess Queen
by Alexis O'Neill, Laura Huliska-Beith (illustrator)

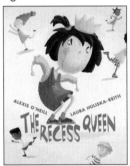

Mean Jean is the recess bully, pushing and dominating the playground. It isn't until a small girl, new to the class, invites Jean to play instead of avoiding her that Mean Jean's behavior turns around. This book is good to use with middle elementary age ESCs.

There is a lot of talk today about bullies and how bullying is not to be tolerated. The flip side of that is that although many of our students do have to deal with genuine mean or bullying behavior of others, many also over-generalize the concept and see many "expected" playground behaviors as bullying. This book works well to show how sometimes children let the rubber chicken get the best of them. They may start out with a "whoopsie" and either not recognize it or let it define them. Whether they identify themselves as Mean Jean or know other children who can be seen as Mean Jean, the rubber chicken can be used to turn the story around.

Questions to ask. What are some of Mean Jean's rubber chicken moments? Does she know how what she is doing makes other people think and feel? Do you think if she was being a Social Detective she might change what she was doing? Why or why not? What were the social cues she missed?

The Worst-Case Scenario Survival Handbook: Middle School
by David Borgenicht, Ben H. Winters, and Robin Epstein; Chuck Gonzales (illustrator)

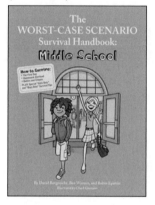

This is a valuable choice for middle school higher social thinking students. This nonfiction how-to book addresses such common subjects as homework, disagreeing with teachers, and dealing with rumors. One section, "How to Survive a Massive Mess-up," is great when introducing the concept of the rubber chicken. The example given is what to do if you mess up on your lines in the school play (minimize the damage, fake it, tease yourself first, and learn from your mistakes), but the concepts can be used in a variety of situations. Here is where I like to talk to the students about my own rubber chicken moments and how I've dealt with them. I ask them to think of other situations they know about that could be rubber chicken moments and how the person involved could deal with it. We do a lot of laughing and saying "That's a good one!" to make the subject light-hearted and fun. We talk about how to repair any damage that may have resulted and how we can avoid it the next time.

Sideways Stories from Wayside School
by Louis Sachar, Julie Brinckloe (illustrator)

This book is a good one to use with late elementary and middle school high social thinking students. Sacher's collection of tales from an imaginary school that was incorrectly constructed is great for a variety of lessons. Wayside School was supposed to have been built as a one-story building with thirty rooms. However, the contractor turned the building plan onto its side and built it thirty stories high with one room on each floor. There is no elevator, and, by the way, there is also no nineteenth floor. Miss Zarves teaches on the nineteenth floor. The

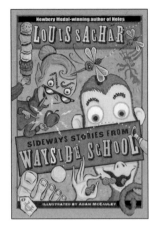

stories, as well as the characters, are just somewhat sideways.

Each chapter in this book is a self-contained story, and each is zany and silly. For example, in Chapter 3, Joe has a unique way of counting. If he is counting objects, he counts out of order (e.g., 4, 7, 1, 3, 9) but always arrives at the right answer. If he is forced to count in order, he can't come up with the correct answer. In Chapter 4, readers meet Sharie, who has the habit of falling asleep in class. One day while she is asleep, Sharie falls out of the window. Thankfully, Louis catches Sharie before she hits the ground. Sharie gets mad at Louis because he woke her up from a good dream by catching her.

Rubber chicken moments are prevalent and blatant in the stories as are expected and unexpected situations and reactions. These short stories also lend themselves well to inferencing opportunities.

14

Size of Problems

|||||||||||||||||||||||||||||||||||||||||||||||||||||||||||||||||||||||||||||||||||||||||||||||||||||||||||||||||||||||||||||||||||||||

Definition

Problems come in sizes, some bigger than others. For example, not doing a homework assignment is more significant than getting the wrong color game piece, but being in a car accident is worse than either. Learning to recognize the size of a problem is the first step in learning to have a reaction that matches the size of that problem. Having a huge reaction to a small problem causes people to have those pesky "uncomfortable thoughts" about you or might even get you in trouble. Plus, how will you react if you come across a big problem in your life if you have already wasted all your big reactions on small problems?

Book Examples

The Chocolate-Covered-Cookie Tantrum
by Deborah Blumenthal, Harvey Stevenson (illustrator)

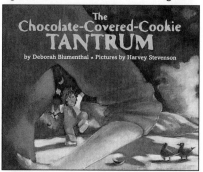

This tale is of a young girl named Sophie who spots a chocolate-covered cookie that another child has. When Sophie asks her mom for the cookie and is told "no," Sophie has a giant tantrum. This tantrum actually metaphorically spins the whole world around. After Sophie goes through her whole tantrum and finally calms down, she goes home with her mom, takes a nap, eats dinner, and is surprised by her own chocolate-covered cookie.

This is an excellent example of having a huge reaction to a small problem. I use this with younger or more beginning social thinkers. I place the numbers 1–5 (1–10 for older or higher-thinkers) in front of the group. We then draw a quick picture of the chocolate-covered cookie and place it somewhere on the line. We make some other pictures of different problems (e.g., a car accident, a hurricane, missing the turn on a drive). We then draw Sophie having the tantrum described in the story and place it where we think it belongs. We draw other pictures of reactions Sophie might have (e.g., calm body, angry face only, running off the face of the earth). We then discuss whether the size of her reaction matched the size of the problem. We also talk about what Sophie could have done to match the problem to the reaction in a better way or more quickly and discuss our own problems and which ones we have a hard time matching with our reactions. It's an introduction to the very big concept of size of problems and one that we revisit frequently.

Questions to ask. How is the mom feeling in the beginning when the mom and Sophie are playing together? What is the mom's body saying when she tells Sophie "no" for the first time? Why is her hand on her hip? What is the mom's face saying when Sophie begins her tantrum? Do you think the mom has seen this behavior before? Who else notices the tantrum? Why is the mom so patient with Sophie? Do you think Sophie's friends would be so patient with Sophie?

When Sophie Gets Angry—Really, Really Angry . . .
by Molly Bang

For use with young or high-emotion students, this story is about a girl who has a squabble with her sister over a stuffed gorilla. When the mom steps in and tells Sophie (a different Sophie than the tantrum Sophie) it is her sister's turn, it's like a volcano erupts from inside of her. Sophie runs and runs and cries and cries, and it takes some time for her emotions to calm down enough so that she can enjoy the outside scenery and then return home.

You can use this book and the tantrum book in conjunction with the *Incredible 5-Point Scale* by Kari Dunn Buron. This resource is a visual way to help students understand and control their emotions. As you read this book, you can have a visual 5-point scale available and put a little game piece "Sophie" on the number the group thinks represents how she is feeling—from 1 for calm and relaxed to 5 for volcano erupting. The group can also use the scale to decide the size of the problem she encountered with her sister and decide if Sophie's reaction matched the same number. The game piece can be moved up and down and the students can show with their own bodies how the different numbers might look. This is only effective with a well-controlled group, however.

Questions to ask. How do you think Sophie felt before the argument? How did her feelings change or stay the same? How did her reaction affect the way her sister and her mom were thinking about her? How could she have behaved differently to keep them thinking about her the way she wanted them to? What are some things Sophie could do to help her move down the stress scale? What makes you climb to a 5? What do you do to move back down the scale?

Alexander and the Terrible, Horrible, No Good, Very Bad Day
by Judith Viorst, Ray Cruz (illustrator)
Poor Alexander! His day is just not going well. Every little thing is going wrong, making for a terrible, horrible, no good, very bad day. We all have days like this.

I use this book with young elementary, high ESC students in the same manner as *When Sophie Gets Angry—Really, Really Angry...* We made up a new Unthinkable (see Chapter 18: Superflex and the Unthinkables) called Snowball Man who makes little things pile up in our brains until they become a big problem. One small problem can become a big problem if we don't address it when it is small.

Questions to ask. How did the day start for Alexander? What are all the problems he identifies? How big is each problem by itself? How did they become a big problem? How big was his reaction? How could Alexander have stopped the snowball from getting too big? Do you ever have days like this? What do you do about your snowball? What would you tell Alexander if you were his friend?

Edwurd Fudwupper Fibbed Big
by Berkeley Breathed
Berkeley Breathed, creator of the *Bloom County* comic strip, has written an amazing story with terrific illustrations. While some of his stories may be useful for ESCs, students with more inference skills will benefit from this thought-provoking tale. You can use this story to analyze characters' body language and facial expressions and make inferences based on the illustrations and background knowledge. Students can identify what

characters are thinking and how they are reacting to other characters' behavior and thoughts.

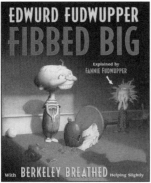

In this particular Breathed story, a young girl adores her older big brother who does not pay much attention to her. In fact, he's a tremendous fibber and tells tall tales about her and everything else. One day, one of his fibs goes a little too far and causes intergalactic troubles. The younger sister, however, saves the day, and Edwurd learns to appreciate her.

When using this story, I have the students spend time looking at and analyzing the illustrations. Breathed has put much more into the story than what appears in the text. This book also presents the opportunity to show students "thought bubbles" as they are included as part of the story. When I use this book to present the size of problems concept, we talk about what size of a problem each of Edwurd's "fibs" represents. For example, when he tells his friends that his sister was born from a dog, it's not a big problem, although it affects how his sister feels. When he tells the fib that Mabel Dill was elected president of Brazil, and she goes there, how big of a problem will that be? And when he tells the fib (that seems like a small fib) that aliens broke the pig, what is the effect of that fib?

Questions to ask. What is Fannie thinking? Why do you think Edwurd makes up stories? What does he hope his friends will think when he tells them Fannie was born from a dog? How does that make Fannie feel? What is Edwurd's body saying when he breaks the pig and gets caught? What might happen to the porcelain pig when the space pig tries to kiss it? Where is Mabel? What happened to her? How did that lie cause a problem for Edwurd now? What does Edwurd feel when fingers get pointed at him? Why did Fannie step in? What does that make Edwurd think and feel? How do you think what happened changed the alien? What does Edwurd think of Fannie now? How does that make her feel?

15

Smart and Wacky Guesses

Definition

We make judgments and predictions all the time about the people and situations around us. We do this based on our past experiences and knowledge. Using our knowledge, we make either "smart guesses," which are good predictions of what might happen, or "wacky guesses," which are based either on our own self-interest or random thoughts. Someone who is proficient at social thinking makes smart guesses on a moment-by-moment basis.

Smart guesses are guesses that make sense, taking into account what knowledge we already have about the people involved, the environment, what's already happened, and social expectations. These guesses are more likely to be accurate (although not always). Wacky guesses are just random guesses that have no logical base in reality. They are rarely accurate and do not help us gather and use important information.

Book Examples

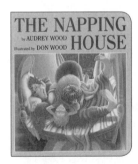

The Napping House
by Audrey Wood, Don Wood (illustrator)

This is a fun book for a preschool or an early elementary school group. In this story, a house is full of sleeping people and creatures. This is a formula book, so it starts with "There is a house, a napping house, where everyone is sleeping," and then adds a line to that sentence on each page. At first, grandma is in the bed, then the boy climbs on top of granny and goes back to sleep, and then the dog climbs on the boy, and then the cat climbs on the dog, and so forth.

When I use this book with students, I scan the pages in the book and crop out everything but the newest addition on that page. I print illustrations of each individual character, laminate them, and attach Velcro. With groups of younger students, we take turns adding the new picture to a flannel board as we read the story. Then, at the end, we try to piece together the story from memory. This is fairly easy to do because each character is smaller than the previous one. To make it a little more challenging, we put the characters in different orders and talk about what might result if that's how the events take place (for example, if the mouse is on the bottom, he might get squished).

This is a good book to work on making smart and wacky guesses. At the beginning of the story, I ask students what they think will happen next. Often at the beginning, the guesses are wackier, and we giggle about our guesses so as not to create anxiety about getting the "wrong" answer. As the book continues and the formula is identified, more "smart" guesses emerge, and we get to pat ourselves on the back (we literally reach our own arm around our own shoulder and pat) as we make smart guesses.

Audrey Wood also wrote *Silly Sally,* which has a similar formula and is great for the same activities.

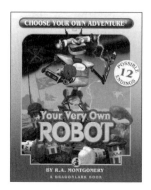

Your Very Own Robot
by R.A. Montgomery

This is one of many Choose Your Own Adventure books, great to use for late elementary and early middle school students who are beginning to make some good inferences and think ahead. In this particular story, you (the reader) inherit a broken-down robot from your scientist parents. After you read a little, you are asked to make a choice. If you do one thing, you turn to a certain page and continue reading. If you choose something else, you turn to a different page and continue. And so the story goes. You create it with your choices.

What is helpful about this series is that it's written at the early chapter book level with fairly large text and simple vocabulary and includes many illustrations. I like to have the students look at the text and think about what might be happening on those pages before we read them together. Then, when we read, we can observe if our guesses were right or if the story went in a different direction than we anticipated. After reading each new scenario, we work together to make a choice, using the information we have gathered and decided on as a group. It's fun to see where our choices take us.

Questions to ask. What choice should we make? How will we decide whose idea we should go with? What should we do if we don't like the outcome? What other directions could the story take? What are some smart and some wacky ideas?

Greeting cards, comics, and joke books

By the preteen years, students who are WISC social thinkers are beginning to develop humor beyond knock-knock jokes. They enjoy humor, they like making humor, and they love making people laugh. They are, however, often hindered by vocabulary (e.g., idioms, dual-meaning words, and other figurative language) and social connectivity (e.g., knowing when someone is laughing because they're having weird or uncomfortable thoughts or when they're laughing because the joke is funny). Greeting cards are great because they present a funny situation that you have to figure out, often a play on words or an amusing social scenario. They're also very short so they don't take a long time to analyze. I can pass out a card or two to every student in a group, and we discuss each one during a Book Chat period. For example, in one Humpty Dumpty was cracked and being taken into an emergency room at "the Mayo Clinic." Inside the card was something to the effect of, "Hope your Easter's all it's cracked up to be." The student analyzing this card immediately understood that the "cracked up" comment was funny because of the crack in Humpty Dumpty. However, he didn't know why "the Mayo Clinic" was funny. I explained that The Mayo Clinic is a real clinic, but also that "mayo" is another word for "mayonnaise," and mayonnaise is made out of...what do you think? The student guessed "eggs" correctly and started laughing. Just a little education on that one, and the whole group enjoyed the laugh!

Comic strips are also good for analyzing social situations. You can use *Calvin and Hobbes* because Calvin is always exhibiting unexpected behavior and misinterpreting social cues. *Peanuts* and *Garfield* are also tried and true staples with many discussion possibilities. Joke books are another fun way to start a group. All of these are more for learning

83

pragmatic language like idioms and double-meanings and not so much for social learning, but they are still great ice-breakers for starting a group.

16

The Social Fake

||||||||||||||||||||||||||||||||||||||||||||||||||||||||||||||||||||||||||||||||||||||||||||||||||||||||||

Definition

We've all done the social fake. It's how we pretend to like that one mom in the PTA who really gets on our nerves or how we survive the holidays with our crazy families. At times we have to "fake" liking someone, being good at something, or showing interest in someone because a social situation calls for it. We do this because we want to be skilled social persons and, more often than not, we do this in social conversations. We don't have to act fascinated with what someone is telling us about his or her life, but we do act like we are interested even if we are not. Doing the social fake is a critical step towards maintaining a friendship or even working well in a group.

Book Examples

How to Be a Friend
by Laurie Krasny Brown and Marc Brown

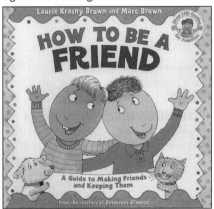

This instructional book is geared towards preschool age students but could be used with students who have moderate social cognitive challenges up through elementary school. It includes many valuable ideas and illustrations that show ways a young person can be a good friend, including joining in, dealing with bullies, and handling arguing.

Questions to ask. You can use this book to introduce flexible thinking with friends. For example, one picture shows two friends working at a table, and one friend says, "This math is hard. I don't get it!" and the other responds, "Try it this way." We talk about what the frustrated friend would and could do. Should he walk away? He doesn't like what they're doing, so why not? What would that make his friend think about him? What should he do instead?

In another picture, two girls are getting their lunch, and one says, "My parents are getting divorced. Please don't tell anyone," and the other friend says, "I promise." We talk about making and keeping secrets and promises. What is a secret we should keep? What is one we shouldn't? What should we do if a friend tells us something and we don't know if we should keep the secret?

Another part of the book is about making up with friends. You can talk with the group about when it's appropriate and helpful to forgive and forget. Why not just leave a friend who has hurt us? When is it worth trying to repair a friendship? What if we are still hurt? How can we act forgiving even if we don't feel it yet? What is it appropriate to forgive but *not* forget? These are all thinking questions that students may not have considered before.

First Grade, Here I Come!
By Nancy Carlson

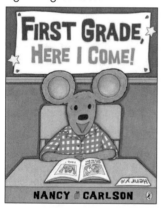

Henry comes home from school after the first day of first grade and seems a little disappointed that it's different than kindergarten. As he describes his day to his mom, though, it seems that he had a flexible brain as he learned a new routine, met new people, and had new adventures. I use this story with young elementary students who may be struggling to handle change or learning how to "fake it" when they don't like how something is going.

Questions to ask. What is Henry thinking about when he first gets home? Why is he thinking about kindergarten? What does Henry's face and body tell you when he gets to first grade and sees his new teacher for the first time? How did Henry make his new friend Oswaldo? In what way did Henry have to "fake it" in first grade? How do you think he felt when he made it through the first day and all the differences he encountered?

I Am a Booger...Treat Me with Respect!
by Julia Cook, Carson Cook (illustrator)

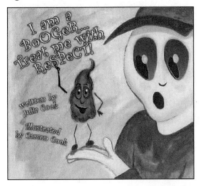

This is one of the best books I've ever run across. It is fun and silly, but best of all, it is blunt. Students with social cognitive disorders like facts and direct information, and this book provides both. Many students have a problem picking their nose! It seems that students with less awareness of the impact of their behavior on others have a particular problem with holding back in this area. This book speaks from the perspective of the booger. It includes good factual information about who the booger is and what he does. "When you breathe in through your nose, the air that you breathe in isn't always clean. Sometimes it has dirt and germs in it. Whenever I see a piece of dirt or a germ inside your nose, I swallow it!" It offers helpful ideas about how to stay healthy and socially appropriate ways to deal with boogers. For example, the book suggests using a "Booger Ghost" (a tissue over your finger) and recommends doing this in private. The booger makes it very clear how gross and unhealthy it is to *eat* him: "When other people see you eat your boogers, it makes them feel sick!"

I never use this book as a reprimand. It's an enjoyable way to make students aware and knowledgeable about this common bad habit. I am also careful not to use it with students who are reinforced by engaging in unexpected behavior to gain the attention of others—it could cause an increase in the behavior I'm trying to eliminate!

Questions to ask. Why is it important to listen to Mr. Booger? What kinds of thoughts can we make people have? How will that affect our relationship with them? When would it be more and less acceptable to pick or scratch inside our nose? In a choir concert on stage? In a classroom? At the dinner table? In our room with friends? Why does it change?

Diary of a Wimpy Kid
by Jeff Kinney

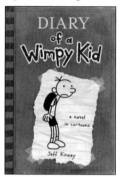

See Chapter 9: Flexible Brain for a synopsis of the book. The premise of *Wimpy Kid* is all about the social fake. Greg just wants to fit in at middle school and has to work hard at it (and isn't always successful). He just happens to be a scrawny, slightly odd boy with nerdy friends. Greg's best friend Rowley is more nerdy than he is, so Greg tries to help his friend blend in. Standing at their lockers, Rowley comes up to Greg and asks "Want to come over to my house and plaayyy?" Greg points out that "I have told Rowley at least a billion times that now that we're in middle school, you're supposed to say 'hang out,' not 'play.' But no matter how many noogies I give him, he always forgets the next time."

The book is written in a way to engage even reluctant readers. It's full of drawings and funny one-liners. Even how the text is formatted alleviates some of the feeling of "serious reading." The book provides some great opportunities to work on inferencing and Social Thinking lessons. For example, in one embedded comic, Greg is shown trying to sell chocolates to neighbors for a fundraiser. The man at the door answers, "Not interested!" and slams the door. The next frame shows Greg's younger brother, a preschooler, trying to sell chocolate at the same house. This time the response is, "How precious!" and the neighbor buys the chocolate. Why the difference? What was the man thinking? How did his response change? This lends itself well to a discussion about how social expectations change over time, and that some things we can get away with when we are younger are not quite as acceptable when we are older. For example, stomping your feet when you don't get your way at two is sort of comical and expected, but seeing that in a twelve-year-old would give other people uncomfortable or weird thoughts about you.

The Worst-Case Scenario Survival Handbook: Middle School
by David Borgenicht, Ben H. Winters, and Robin Epstein; Chuck Gonzales (illustrator)

As described in Chapter 13: Rubber Chicken Moments, this is a wonderful how-to guide to use with groups about surviving middle school, covering

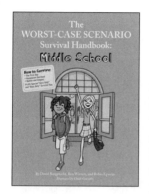

subjects such as fixing a problem with a teacher and surviving changing in the locker room. It's full of funny examples and illustrations to keep students engaged. It's a short read and can be incorporated into a variety of Social Thinking lessons with middle school groups. Insightful tips are offered throughout the book; for example, "Be aware. Slow nodding says, 'I'm listening,' and signals that you're taking your teacher seriously. Too-fast nodding says, 'Okay, I get it, enough already!'" When you get to this tip, students can practice their nod speed.

In the section "How to survive a massive mess-up," tip number two is "Fake it. No matter how much you feel like collapsing in tears, keep playing (or cheering, or acting) with a smile. Freaking out will tell the world that this *is* a big deal. If you stay calm, they may never know." The discussion is specific, clear, and definitely useful for students with social cognitive challenges who tend to "freak out" about small problems. It includes one section specifically geared for boys and another for girls. What works well is to read sections from the book addressing the challenges that students in your group are currently experiencing in their lives.

17

Social Wondering

||||||||||||||||||||||||||||||||||||||||||||||||||||||||||||||||||||||||||||||||||||||||||||||||||||||||||||||||||||||||||||||||||||||||

Definition

This takes the skill of thinking of others to a deeper level. Social wondering means knowing about someone or a social situation and wondering "What if this" and "What if that?" What will happen if I make this choice? What will happen if those kids do that? What will I do? What will be the impact? We also use social wondering when we talk to other people. We wonder about them and their lives. What do they want to talk about? What did they do this weekend? Then, social wondering transcends into action. We use our social wondering to make smart guesses about how what we do or say will affect the thoughts and feelings of others.

Book Examples

Glad Monster, Sad Monster
by Ed Emberley and Anne Miranda

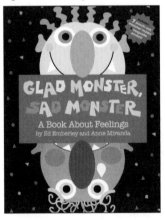

This is a great book to use to introduce thinking of others and their feelings to early and young social thinkers. It is a simple picture book with alternating pages about different colored monsters, what they are doing, and how it is making them feel. "The yellow monster says, 'Opening birthday presents, playing ball, slurping ice cream, and dancing with my friend make me glad.'" Other emotions that are expressed include anger, sadness, worry, and silliness.

The book also has monster face punch-outs of each of the monsters' faces with instructions like "Put on the angry red monster mask. Say what makes you angry."

Questions to ask. When I have used this book in a preschool group, as we read it, I ask questions such as, "What made the monster feel angry? What would you do if you saw a friend angry?" I then return later in the story to the same monster and ask, "Do you remember what made red monster angry?" to work on retrieving previously learned material. We then each take a mask and say, "I feel angry/sad/happy when…" I also ask members of the group to remember what made their friends feel a certain way. "Jamie, do you remember what Alex said that made him feel angry?"

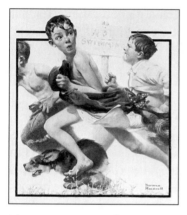

Artworks of Norman Rockwell

These are not books for reading, but analyzing Norman Rockwell paintings has been a valuable tool with my groups for analyzing characters' intentions and underlying meanings as well as for understanding social rules and situations. Many of his paintings depict an entire social scene. Some are more appropriate to show a social group than others, so you have to pick and choose. But when you find a good one, it's great to use with your groups. One favorite is *No Swimming* (1921). This is a picture of some boys running, half naked and wet, away from something. A sign says, "No swimming." More often than not, social thinking students misinterpret the scene and think the kids are running toward the water. I use leading questions to help them recognize that the boys are already wet and they are looking behind

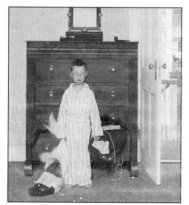

them while they run. What do you think happened? Why are they running? Who do you think they are looking for over their shoulders?

Another good painting to use is *The Discovery* (1956) which is of a little boy with an almost horrified expression, holding a red suit and white beard in front of an open dresser drawer. What does the boy hold? Where did he find it? What is he thinking about? What does his face say? What did he find out? What might happen next? What might his dad say to him? How would you feel?

What you can do with these pictures is tell the students to look and not say anything while they look at the picture. You can then ask each student to mention one thing he or she observes about the picture. They are allowed to share only one thing, which promotes patience and a flexible brain. They have to build upon what the others say to figure out the whole story. Once students begin to present their observations and some of the story of the picture begins to emerge, you can ask leading questions to help them decipher the rest of the meaning. It's fascinating to see what parts of the stories they miss.

Mars Needs Moms!
by Berkeley Breathed

Appropriate for older elementary and higher social thinking students, *Mars Needs Moms!* begins with a boy named Milo being tired of his mom asking him to do chores and eat his vegetables. When he gets in trouble and is sent to his room without supper, he yells to his mother, "I sure don't see what's so special about mothers!" This hurts his mother's feelings (the invaluable illustration on this page can be the basis for a discussion about inferences). That night, Milo's mom is kidnapped by Martians, and Milo sneaks onboard the spaceship. Milo learns a great lesson when they land on Mars!

As with any Berkeley Breathed book, the illustrations in this story lend themselves to discussions about social wondering and inferences.

Questions to ask. What is Milo looking at? What does that mean he is thinking about? What does his mom's body language say when Milo takes out the trash? Why was Milo's mom unhappy when he painted his sister? What does his mom's body say when Milo tells her he doesn't know what's so special about mothers? What does it mean when the book says she closed the door very, very slowly? What is the alien trying to do with the coffee cup and the fishing pole? Why did the Martians come to kidnap moms? What would have happened to Milo's mom if the aliens didn't get her a helmet? Why do you think she gave Milo her helmet? What does his dad know about what happened in the night when they return the next morning?

18

Superflex and the Unthinkables

IIIIIIIIIIIIIIIIIIIIIIIIIIIIIIIIIIIIIIIIIIIIIIIIIIIIIIIIIIIIIIIIIIIIIIIIIIIIIIIIIIIIIIIIIIIIIIIIIIIIIIIIIIIIIIIIIIIIIIIIIIIIIIIIIIIIIIIIIIIIIIIIIIIIIIIII

Definition

Drawing upon many of the students' interest in superheroes, Stephanie Madrigal (a colleague of Michelle Garcia Winner) created the social superhero Superflex (Madrigal and Winner, 2008). He battles a set of evil villains called the Unthinkables, social villains who disrupt good social behavior and prevent us from being effective social thinkers. By reading about Superflex, students learn strategies to defeat the team of Unthinkables living inside of everyone's brains. Using these characters, students start to identify and relate to who is on their team and how they can use their own personal Superflex to lay the Unthinkables to rest.

Following is a list of books that complement the introduction and instruction of the Superflex curriculum as well as some of the Unthinkable characters. Some of these Unthinkables were designed by our staff; most of them are the original set (used with permission). These materials can be used in a Book Chat to go together with a certain topic or just for fun.

Book Examples

Unthinkable	Books
Rock Brain *I make people get stuck on their ideas.*	*Superflex Takes on Rock Brain and the Team of Unthinkables* by Stehanie Madrigal *Beatrice Doesn't Want To* by Laura Numeroff and Lynn Munsinger

Unthinkable	Books

D.O.F.
(Destroyer of Fun)

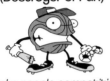

I make people competitive in a mean way.

You're a Good Sport, Miss Malarkey
by Judy Finchler

How to Lose All Your Friends
by Nancy Carlson

Topic Twistermeister

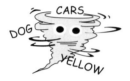

I make people jump off topic.

My Mouth Is a Volcano!
by Julia Cook and Carrie Hartman

One Sided Sid

I get people to only talk about themselves.

I'm The Biggest Thing in the Ocean
by Kevin Sherry

My Mouth Is a Volcano!
by Julia Cook

Little Miss Chatterbox
by Roger Hargreaves

Unwonderer

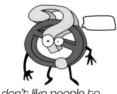

I don't like people to wonder about others.

Watch Out!
by Jan Fearnley

Unthinkable	Books

Body Snatcher

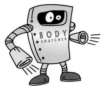

I move people's bodies away from the group.

Beatrice Doesn't Want To
by Laura Numeroff and Lynn Munsinger

Worry Wall

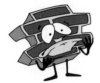

I make people worry too much.

Scaredy Squirrel books
by Melanie Watt

There's an Alligator Under My Bed
by Mercer Mayer

Silly Billy
by Anthony Browne

Energy Hare-y

I give people too much energy.

Some Kids Just Can't Sit Still!
by Sam Goldstein

Why Can't Jimmy Sit Still?
by Sandra L. Tunis

Sit Still!
by Nancy Carlson

Howard B. Wigglebottom Learns to Listen
by Howard Binkow and Susan F. Cornelison

Space Invader

I get people to invade others' personal space.

Beatrice Doesn't Want To
by Laura Numeroff and Lynn Munsinger

Hunter's Best Friend at School
by Laura Malone Elliott and Lynn Munsinger

Personal Space Camp
by Julia Cook

Unthinkable	Books
Grump Grumpaniny *I put people in grumpy moods.*	*Beatrice Doesn't Want To* by Laura Numeroff and Lynn Munsinger *Grumpy Bird* by Jeremy Tankard *The Pout-Pout Fish* by Deborah Diesen *I'm Bored* by Christine Schneider *Mr. Grumpy* by Roger Hargreaves
Glassman 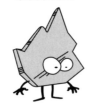 *I make people have huge reactions.*	*Superflex Takes on Glassman and the Team of Unthinkables* by Stehanie Madrigal and Michelle Garcia Winner *How to Take the Grrrr Out of Anger* by Elizabeth Verdick and Marjorie Lisovskis *Mad Isn't Bad: A Child's Book About Anger* by Michaelene Mundy *Don't Sweat the Small Stuff for Teens: Simple Ways to Keep Your Cool in Stressful Times* by Richard Carlson
WasFunnyOnce *I get people to use humor at the wrong time.*	*Hunter's Best Friend at School* by Laura Malone Elliott and Lynn Munsinger *That's Not Funny!* by Adrian Johnson *Mr. Funny* by Roger Hargreaves

Unthinkable	Books

Brain Eater

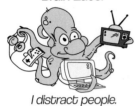

I distract people.

Mr. Daydream
by Roger Hargreaves

Mean Jean

I get people to act mean and bossy.

Bootsie Barker Bites
by Barbara Bottner

The Recess Queen
by Alexis O'Neill

Bossy Bear
by David Horvath

The Enforcer

I want to make everybody follow all the rules.

Little Miss Bossy
by Roger Hargreaves

Franklin Is Bossy (Franklin Series)
by Paulette Bourgeois and Brenda Clark

Snowball Man

I let little problems stack up until they're a big problem.

Alexander and the Terrible, Horrible, No Good, Very Bad Day
by Judith Viorst

Unthinkable	Books

Sell-Fish

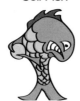

I don't like to share.

Bossy Bear
by David Horvath

It's Mine!
by Leo Lionni

Int-Erupter

I interrupt when other people are talking.

We Listen: We Don't Interrupt
by Donna Luck

Tattle Taylor

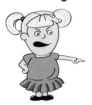

I tattle on my friends about unimportant matters.

A Bad Case of Tattle Tongue
by Julia Cook

Don't Squeal Unless It's a Big Deal: A Tale of Tattletales
by Jeanie Franz Ransom

The Blaminator

I blame other people for everything wrong that happens to me.

It's Not My Fault!
by Nancy L. Carlson

19

Thinking About You/Just Me

|||||||||||||||||||||||||||||||||||||||||||||||||||||||||||||||||||||||||||||||||||||||||||||||||||||||||||||||||||||||||||||||||||||||||||||||

Definition

Most of the time we are expected to be a Thinking of You person. This means we recognize that our behavior affects the people around us, and we strive to change how we act in such a way as to keep other people thinking about us the way we want them to. There are times when it is acceptable to be a Just Me person, focusing on our own needs alone. For students, this happens when they get time all to themselves like when they read or play a video game in their room and are not expected to be doing anything for anyone else (chores, homework, etc.). However, even then they have to think about others because if they make a lot of noise or a mess, they could impact the feelings and thoughts of others. Even when they are home and want to watch TV after finishing homework, a Thinking of You person does not just change the channel if someone else is already watching TV. That is what a Just Me person would do. A Thinking of You person might ask if the other person wants to watch something different or might sit down and watch what that person is already watching or might simply strike up a conversation.

Book Examples

Join In and Play
by Cheri J. Meiners, M.Ed.

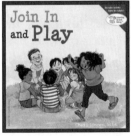

This book comes from a series of *Learning to Get Along®* books that deal with a variety of "friendly" behaviors like listening, being polite, and sharing. This particular book teaches the basics of cooperating, sharing, making friends, and thinking of others. In the beginning, the girl is playing on her own in a sort of Just Me manner. Then she wants to go out and be with friends. The book tells in simple ways how she has to behave in a Thinking of You manner to make and keep those friends. For example, she has to smile and say hello. She can ask a question to start a conversation. She can ask or offer to play. She can ask a grown-up if she needs help. And so forth.

This is great for preschool or early elementary age beginning social thinking students. The "rules" are clear and direct. The illustrations are descriptive, too. For example, in one spread, a boy and a girl had clearly been playing blocks together, but the illustration shows the girl walking away with a "snotty" demeanor and the boy looking on, baffled. It's a great place to stop and work on thinking with eyes and brain and inferencing what might have happened and how the characters are feeling.

Questions to ask. In this picture, who is Thinking About You? Who is Just Me? What is the girl looking at and seeing outside her window? What is she thinking? How did the girl become Thinking About You after being Just Me? When the girl walks away with the LEGOs, what are her friends thinking about her?

If You Give a Mouse a Cookie
by Laura Numeroff, Felicia Bond (illustrator)

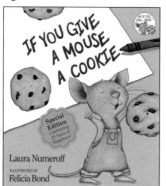

A demanding mouse runs a young boy ragged trying to fulfill his demands. From eating cookies to cutting hair to drawing, the boy is left to clean up after the energetic mouse.

This formula-based book is great for younger students. After the first few pages, students should be able to predict that the mouse will want something new. Throughout the story, the mouse makes demands on the boy and appears unaware of the effect this has on the boy's demeanor and emotional state. Compare the first page where the boy offers the mouse a cookie (the boy is all smiles and hands over the cookie willingly) to the last page where the boy sits on the floor, eyes and head down, surrounded by a mess. The mouse looks quite content, but how does the boy feel?

Questions to ask. How do you know what the mouse/boy is feeling…? What about each of their bodies tells you that? Why does the boy help the mouse? When the mouse is cleaning, what are his intentions? *(He intends to help the boy.)* What is the reality? *(It causes more mess for the boy to clean up after.)* Who is being Just Me? Who is being Thinking of You? How do you think the boy will feel the next time he has an interaction with the mouse? How will his feelings change, and what might he do differently?

This book goes well with *The Cat in the Hat* by Dr. Seuss. In that story, a large cat comes over when the parents are gone and tries to "have fun" with the kids, but his fun makes a mess of the house and causes a lot of stress for the kids. Many of the same principles can be used with that book. In addition, there is a whole series of these "If You Give a... a ..." books by Numeroff, all of which can be used to emphasize the same ideas.

If Everybody Did
by Jo Ann Stover
This is a book of glaring examples of what might happen if everybody engaged in mildly annoying or distracting behavior. The book starts with, "When there's only one, that's just somebody, but when there's one and one and one and more, that's everybody!" It then goes into various examples of what would happen if everybody did things like jump in the mud or make a big splash. On the left side of each page is a line drawing of one person engaging in the behavior; the right side has a picture of a lot of people engaging in the behavior and what that might look like. This can be used with younger, high social thinking students or even students who are a little older, up to later elementary school, who are more challenged in their social thinking abilities.

You can use this book as an introduction to Just Me/Thinking About You. After reading the book, the group can try to come up with additional suggestions that are more realistic to the group like taking shoes off, picking noses, and interrupting. If you have a more compliant group, you can ask them to act out what it would look like. For groups that need more structure, you can have students make their own line drawing pictures and then share them with each other. You can make it fun and silly while illustrating how distracting and hard it would be for the group to run if "everybody" did this or that.

Questions to ask. How do the actions on the left make other people feel? How about the right? How do some of the actions on the right make things more difficult for other people? How can they sometimes be unsafe? How can they change the way people are thinking about you? Can you think of other things that could fit in this book on the left and on the right?

The Giving Tree
by Shel Silverstein

Shel Silverstein is a great poet and author to use for helping students work on developing a good sense of humor. His poetry books, parables, and fables are witty, endearing, and sometimes irreverent, perfect for socially developing students, especially boys. In this Silverstein book, which I like to use with late elementary school and early middle school students, a boy grows up with a tree. Over the years, the boy has times when he seems unhappy and wants something, and the tree gives it to him. When the boy is happy, the tree is happy. However, it becomes more and more difficult to keep the boy happy, and the tree has to give more and more (his apples, his branches, his trunk) until there is nothing left but a stump. Then, the boy, now an old man, comes to rest, and the tree, now a stump, offers a place to sit. The man rests, and the tree is happy. Is it healthy to give-give-give or take-take-take? Is being either way really going to bring happiness? How can we find that balance in our lives? Why is it important?

Questions to ask. When is the boy a Just Me person? When does he show some Thinking About You? Who is the "you" in this story? How does the tree show it is a Thinking About You individual? How could the tree have helped the boy *become* more of a Thinking About You person? Does this relationship work? For the boy? For the tree? What effect does their relationship have on other people?

The Missing Piece Meets the Big O
by Shel Silverstein

In this Silverstein book, a pie-shaped "piece" is looking for its missing piece to make it whole. It tries to attract potential suitors in a variety of ways to no avail. In the end, it comes across a whole, the Big O, but the Big O doesn't have a missing piece, so it doesn't need the missing piece. The Big O tells the missing piece that he can become whole, too. The missing piece then starts forcing itself to flop along, and, as it does, its edges begin to round. Eventually, the missing piece is its own Big O. It then meets the other Big O and they roll off together.

I use this book to introduce, in a light-hearted way, the subject of dating. Some students with social cognitive difficulties think that there is just some magic and people match up together and all's well. They get discouraged or don't try at all. They can be taught that dating is a lot about trying on potential mates to see if they fit. There is a lot of rejection and changing, and that is all normal. In addition, it's important to work on our own sharp edges as we search in the hopes that we can become our own Big O as we find a good match.

Questions to ask. Why was it important for the missing piece to find someone to fit with? What does the Big O teach the missing piece? How? How can you see yourself as a missing piece and/or the Big O? At what different times and places in your life are you either one? When is it beneficial for you to smooth out sharp edges and when is it okay to stay pie-shaped?

20

Thinking with Eyes

‖‖‖

Definition

We show what we're thinking about largely by what we're looking at. If we're looking at our watch, we're probably thinking about what time it is but also if we're going to be late somewhere. People often show they are keeping their brain in the group when they think about the speaker with their eyes. Teachers often show who they want to talk to by looking at a specific student, even if they don't call the student's name. When we think with our eyes, we can also see how people feel and start to make better predictions about what might happen next.

Book Examples

The Red Book
by Barbara Lehman

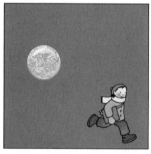

This story is told through pictures only (no text), and is best for middle to late elementary school students. A girl finds a red book on the way to school. When she opens it at school, on the pages she sees a boy who is also looking at a red book. In *his* red book, he is looking at her looking in *her* red book. They see each other! On the way home from school, she buys a bunch of balloons and floats away, but her red book falls out of her hands to the ground. The boy in the book sees the girl's book fall and is sad. But, he receives a surprise.

The goal is to get the students to figure out the story without text. This takes a lot of thinking with both their eyes and brains and using inferencing skills because they have to look at body language and what's happening in the environment, make predictions about what might happen next, and understand the story's outside-of-reality possibilities.

Questions to ask. What do you think the girl found (before finding out it is a book)? What does the girl think about during class? What are her classmates thinking about? How do you know? What are the boy and the girl thinking when they each realize the other one can see them in the book? What would you think? What do you think she will do? What is the boy in the book thinking when he realizes the girl's book does not show her anymore? As you look at the last page, what do you think will happen next?

David Wiesner has written other similar books, such as *Flotsam, Tuesday, Sector 7,* and *June 29, 1999*. All have little to no text, and each story depends on using the illustrations to make inferences.

He Came with the Couch
by David Slonim

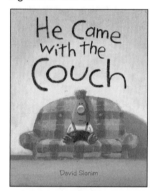

A family needs a new couch. They have a hard time finding one, but when they find the right one, it comes with a bonus—a creature sitting on the couch. "He came with the couch" the author writes. This creature (you're not sure if it is a doll or real until about halfway through) just sits there and doesn't move. The family can't get him *off* the couch to use it! They try an assortment of tricks, but to the delight of the little girl (and the chagrin of the parents), he's just stuck there. One day, the girl falls out of a tree, and, in a split second, the creature is off the couch and throwing the couch out the window to save the girl. Guess he wasn't so bad after all.

This is a great story told with vivid illustrations and very little text and is a good choice for working on inferencing skills. The whole story culminates with one two-page spread where the reader sees only the creature's hands out the window, the couch having been thrown out, and the little girl falling. Throughout the book, it's important to have the students identify how the girl and the parents are feeling about the creature because it will then be more meaningful when you come to the spread with the girl falling.

Questions to ask. Use your eyes to look at all the things in this picture (Larry's 24 hour Rummage). What do you see? What do the different items mean? Where do you think they came from? What is the girl thinking about when she is looking at "him" in the back of the truck? What is the mom thinking about when she is sitting at the kitchen table? What about the dad? What is the mom thinking when she is looking at "him" when they are watching the movie? Look at the picture (of "him" throwing the couch out the window) and explain what each part of the picture is and what it means. What is the girl thinking afterwards? What is "he" thinking? The parents? How have the family's feelings changed?

21

Whopping Topic Change

||||||||||||||||||||||||||||||||||||||||||||||||||||||||||||||||||||||||||||||||||||||||||||||||||||||||||||||||||||||||||||||||||||||

Definition

This is when someone cannot figure out how one comment relates to something else that was just said. The conversational partner seems to have just said something unrelated to the current flow of the conversation, which gives the other person weird or uncomfortable thoughts. For example: Student 1 says: "I saw a great movie this weekend." Student 2 says: "Did you know the earth is 93 million miles from the sun?" This often happens in groups when a student asks a question that has absolutely nothing to do with the activity at hand. When students engage in "whopping topic changes" (WTCs), I might respond by saying, "I'm confused. We were just talking about such-and-such. I'm not sure how your question connects to what we were discussing." Sometimes, students can explain the connection, but because they did not do so when they made the statement, I give them the chance to do it now. If they can connect the question to what we were discussing, we can address it. If they can't make the connection, I ask them to "put it in their pocket" until we get to a break. One trick of using language well is to explain how your thinking connects to another person's thinking. This is called narrative language, and it is a critical skill for written expression.

Book Examples

My Mouth Is a Volcano!
by Julia Cook, Carrie Hartman (illustrator)

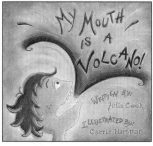

Louis seems to have a volcano in his mouth. Whenever someone is talking and Louis thinks of something he wants to say, he just can't control it. His tummy rumbles and grumbles, his words wiggle and jiggle, and then his tongue pushes them out like a volcano. Louis gets into trouble for interrupting his friends, teacher, and family, but he doesn't understand why this is a problem. Then, when he is giving a talk in front of the class, two of his classmates interrupt *him,* and he is irritated that they took away his time and attention. His mom kindly points out that that is how other people feel when Louis's volcano erupts. She gives him some good ideas on how to control his volcano, and he learns a valuable lesson.

I use this book with early to middle elementary school students with fairly high social thinking abilities. There are some great examples of WTCs as well as of simply monopolizing the conversation. In addition, the author does an effective job of making the unexpected behavior of talking out external to the child. It's "my volcano's fault." I love this because it takes the burden off the student and puts it on something else. His mom's advice for Louis is excellent. She tells him that the next time his "important words" try to come out of his mouth, he should attempt to bite down hard and not let them out, and then take a deep breath and push the words out his nose. When it's his turn to talk, he can take a deep breath and breathe them all back in and say them. The excellent illustrations give the students concrete images to think about and imagine as they try to gain control over their thoughts.

Questions to ask. How does Louis feel when he waits so long for his turn to talk? What is Louis thinking about during story time? How do you know? What are the other students thinking about? How do you know? What thoughts did Louis have about his friends who interrupted him during his "Student Star" poster share? Who is Louis thinking about at the dinner table when his sister is talking? How do you know? How will controlling his volcano change the way his friends think about him?

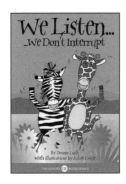

We Listen...We Don't Interrupt
by Donna Luck, Juliet Doyle (illustrator)
Gino and Zelda are best friends, but Zelda has a problem listening to her friend when he wants to say something. Throughout the story, Zelda cuts Gino off and doesn't listen to what he says. In the end, Zelda almost misses out on Gino's birthday party because he wouldn't listen to her!

This is a great book to use with younger elementary age students or those who are just beginning to understand the concept of listening with your eyes and using your brain when communicating with others.

Questions to ask. How did it make Gino feel when Zelda didn't listen to him? What kinds of thoughts did he have? What was Gino thinking about? Do you think some giraffes might have stopped trying? Why or why not? How do you think Zelda would have felt if she missed the party? What can Zelda do the next time someone tries to talk to her and she begins to think about something else?

Sideways Stories from Wayside School
by Louis Sachar

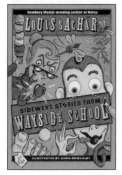

Dana is covered in mosquito bites. However, it's time to do math. Dana is too distracted by her mosquito bites. Ron is tired. Terrence is hungry. Todd says he's "too stupid." These are all random thoughts that seem to have nothing to do with math! Mrs. Jewls gets creative and uses Dana's mosquito bites to teach math. By the end, the bites don't even itch anymore. (See Chapter 13: Rubber Chicken Moments for a more detailed summary of this book.)

This story about Dana, like all the chapters in this book, is silly. Much of the book itself is a series of whopping topic changes. The book offers many opportunities to point out to students how some of the wacky events in the stories are funny on the page but in real life would cause people to have weird or uncomfortable thoughts. For example, if you were talking to a friend about the football game this weekend, and he started talking about the diameter of Saturn, it might cause you to feel uncomfortable and not inclined to want to hang out with him again.

There are several Wayside books, and any one of them can be used to discuss Whopping Topic Change and any of a number of Social Thinking concepts.

22

Reading Comprehension and Social Thinking Goal Ideas

||||||||||||||||||||||||||||||||||||||||||||||||||||||||||||||||||||||||||||||||||||||||||||||||||||||||||||||||||||||||||||||||||||||||||||

When you are developing goals that take into account educational standards as well as social thinking, you can review your state's educational standards as adopted by your state education board. Most of these standards will overlap and resemble those of other states. Although national standards have not been set, similar educational standards have been adopted by most states, at least in the core content areas of reading, writing, and math. For example, in Washington state, the Essential Academic Learning Requirement (EALR) 2 for Reading in Grade 3 is "The student understands the meaning of what is read. Component: 2.2. Understand and apply knowledge of text components to comprehend text. 2.2.3. Understand story elements." *(Online Grade Level Standards and Resources Reading, 2010).* In Texas for Grade 3, it is "110.5. English Language Arts and Reading (11) Reading/text structures/ literary concepts. The student analyzes the characteristics of various types of texts. The student is expected to: (I) identify the importance of the setting to a story's meaning (1-3); and (J) recognize the story problem(s) or plot (1-3)." *(Texas Essential Knowledge and Skills for English Language Arts and Reading, 2010)* And in Maine, "R–3–4: Demonstrate initial understanding of elements of literary texts by… R–3–4.1 Identifying or describing character(s), setting, problem/solution, major events, or plot, as appropriate to text" *(New England Common Assessment Program, 2010).* All three states have a standard that relates to identifying and utilizing story elements but have different ways of expressing that objective.

In addition to taking standards into account, other components contribute to a well-written goal. First, consider the student's present level of performance and use that as the starting place. The end will be determined by when you plan to reassess progress and how fast you think the student can achieve that goal. Most goals in the education field target progress for a year, while in a clinical setting it can vary from three months to a year.

Once you have the start and end points, the goal should be written in a clear and understandable way. It should pass the "Stranger Test," meaning that a stranger who is unfamiliar with the student could understand it. This is especially important when a variety of teachers or therapists deliver instruction to the student. The goal should also be positively stated. It should tell what the student is going to *do*, not what the student *won't do*. For example, "Not hitting" is not a behavior, but "Using words to express frustration during a conflict" is positively stated. Finally, the goal needs to be measurable, and it should be a measurement that makes sense. Goals that say something like "the student will engage in a two-way conversation 80% of the time" is not practical.

More educators are becoming familiar with the SMART method of developing good goals. This stands for **S**pecific (clear descriptions), **M**easurable (must be able to *count* or *observe* it), **A**ction words (must be able to *do* it), **R**ealistic and relevant (based on needs of that student), and **T**ime-related (clear start and end points).

Here is an example of a poorly written goal from an IEP: Student will improve his behavior by keeping hands to himself, maintaining body basics, and completing tasks at a level appropriate to his peer group. Criteria: 80% accuracy, 4 out of 5 opportunities.

Three separate goals are in this example and none are defined. And how will they measure it to 80%?

Here is a better alternative that uses one of the components: Student will improve his circle time attentiveness by maintaining a calm body (eyes looking at speaker, hands to self, body with the group, appropriate voice tone), improving from having a calm body for an average of two minutes to having a calm body for ten minutes, measured at the beginning of the circle time for three consecutive data-taking days.

Social Thinking and Reading Comprehension Goal Ideas
The following is a list of possible goals that combine both reading

comprehension strategies with social thinking expectations. This is not an exhaustive or all-compassing list but merely some suggestions for how to combine the academic and social cognitive needs of a particular student. You can analyze and modify these goals to fit the needs of the particular student and evaluate them over time to see if they measure the progress you want to see in that student. Each reading comprehension strategy presented here includes three possible Social Thinking vocabulary goals and a goal for each of the ILAUGH components listed below.

Reading Comprehension Strategy:
Goal Ideas for Generating and Responding to Essential Questions

Keeping Brain in the Group
When listening and reading along to an oral story at Student's social cognitive level, Student will demonstrate he or she is keeping his or her brain in the group by answering and asking questions with on-topic responses, improving from X out of 5 to 4 out of 5 in each session on three consecutive data days.

Rubber Chicken Moments
When listening and reading along to an oral story at Student's social cognitive level, Student will demonstrate knowledge of social mishaps by identifying them in stories, improving from X out of 5 to 4 out of 5 in each session on three consecutive data days.

Smart and Wacky Guesses
When listening and reading along to an oral story at Student's social cognitive level, Student will make both smart and wacky guesses through asking and answering questions, improving from X out of 5 to 4 out of 5 in each session on three consecutive data days.

I = Initiation of Language
When listening and reading along to an oral story at Student's social cognitive level, Student will volunteer an answer to an indirect question (e.g., a question presented to the whole group) or make an unsolicited, on-topic comment, improving initiation of language from making X comments to making X comments in a fifteen minute listening time on each of three consecutive days.

L = Listening with Eyes and Brain
When listening and reading along to an oral story at Student's social cognitive level, Student will ask and answer questions that demonstrate thinking with eyes and brain (e.g., "I see that person is..." or "Why are they ...?"), improving listening with eyes and brain from X out of 5 to 4 out of 5 responses in each session on three consecutive data days.

A = Abstract/Inferential Language
When listening and reading along to an oral story at Student's social cognitive level, Student will generate social thinking questions or statements that demonstrate inferencing (e.g., "I think they are... because [observation]" or "He wants to ...because [observation]"), improving abstract and inferential language skills from X out of 5 to 4 out of 5 in each session on three consecutive data days.

U = Understanding Perspective
When listening and reading along to an oral story at Student's social cognitive level, Student will generate social thinking questions or statements that demonstrate understanding perspective (e.g., "She is thinking/feeling..." or "I think the author meant/did that because..."), improving from X out of 5 to 4 out of 5 in each session on three consecutive data days.

G = Gestalt Processing/Getting the Big Picture
When listening and reading along to an oral story at Student's social cognitive level, Student will generate social thinking questions or statements that demonstrate gestalt processing (e.g., "I think the story means..." or answers "What is the main idea" questioning), improving from X out of 5 to 4 out of 5 in each session on three consecutive data days.

H = Humor and Human Relatedness
When listening and reading along to an oral story at Student's social cognitive level, Student will generate social thinking questions or statements that demonstrate humor and human relatedness (e.g., "That's funny because..." or "Those characters..."), improving from X out of 5 to 4 out of 5 in each session on three consecutive data days.

Reading Comprehension Strategy:
Goal Ideas for Making Predictions

Social Wondering
When listening and reading along to an oral story at Student's social cognitive level, Student will demonstrate knowledge of social wondering by making predictions (e.g., I wonder if he will...), improving from X out of 5 "smart" predictions to 4 out of 5 in each session on three consecutive data days.

Smart and Wacky Guesses
When listening and reading along to an oral story at Student's social cognitive level, Student will make both smart and wacky guesses through making predictions, improving from X out of 5 "smart" predictions to 4 out of 5 responses in each session on three consecutive data days.

Rubber Chicken Moments
When listening and reading along to an oral story at Student's social cognitive level responses, Student will demonstrate knowledge of social mishaps by making predictions about them (e.g., "I think he's going to..."), improving from X out of 5 to 4 out of 5 responses in each session on three consecutive data days.

I = Initiation of Language
When listening and reading along to an oral story at Student's social cognitive level, Student will volunteer at least one prediction in a group setting, improving initiation of language from initiating X predictions to initiating X predictions in a fifteen minute listening time in each of three consecutive days.

L = Listening with Eyes and Brain
When listening and reading along to an oral story at Student's social cognitive level, Student will make predictions that demonstrate thinking with eyes and brain (e.g., "I think they will...because I see..." or "I think there will be...because I know that..."), improving listening with eyes and brain from X out of 5 to 4 out of 5 in one session on three consecutive data days.

A = Abstract/Inferential Language

When listening and reading along to an oral story at Student's social cognitive level, Student will make predictions that demonstrate inferencing (e.g., "I think they will… because…," "She wants to … because…," or "They might… because that means…"), improving abstract and inferential language skills from X out of 5 to 4 out of 5 in each session on three consecutive data days.

U = Understanding Perspective

When listening and reading along to an oral story at Student's social cognitive level, Student will make predictions that demonstrate understanding perspective (e.g., "He might…because he is thinking/feeling…" or "I think it might…because the author…"), improving from X out of 5 to 4 out of 5 in each session on three consecutive data days.

G = Gestalt Processing/Getting the Big Picture

When listening and reading along to an oral story at Student's social cognitive level, Student will make predictions that demonstrate gestalt processing (e.g., "They already… so they might…" or answers "What might happen in the next chapter/book knowing what you know about…" questioning), improving from X out of 5 to 4 out of 5 in each session on three consecutive data days.

H = Humor and Human Relatedness

When listening and reading along to an oral story at Student's social cognitive level, Student will make predictions that demonstrate humor and human relatedness (e.g., "They think/feel…so they might…" or "He likes…so he might…"), improving from X out of 5 to 4 out of 5 in each session on three consecutive data days.

Reading Comprehension Strategy:
Goal Ideas for Making Connections

Flexible Brain

When listening and reading along to an oral story at Student's social cognitive level, Student will make text connections (i.e., text-to-text, text-to-self, text-to-world) while demonstrating a flexible brain (e.g., connecting to more than one genre, allowing friends to disagree, or accepting corrections), from initiating X connections to initiating X connections in a fifteen minute listening time on each of three consecutive days.

Thinking About You/Just Me
When listening and reading along to an oral story at Student's social cognitive level, Student will make text connections (i.e., text-to-text, text-to-self, text-to-world) that demonstrate Thinking About You/Just Me (e.g., "I see she is being Thinking About You which makes me think of…" or "That character must be a Just Me right now which is how I feel when…"), from X out of 5 to 4 out of 5 in each session on three consecutive data days.

People (or Friend) Files
When listening and reading along to an oral story at Student's social cognitive level, Student will make text connections (i.e., text-to-text, text-to-self, text-to-world) that demonstrate knowledge of friend files (e.g., "Jason knows that Sally doesn't like peanuts because he learned that in the last chapter."), from X out of 5 to 4 out of 5 in each session on three consecutive data days.

I = Initiation of Language
When listening and reading along to an oral story at Student's social cognitive level, Student will volunteer text connections (i.e., text-to-text, text-to-self, text-to-world) in a group setting, improving initiation of language from initiating X connections to initiating X connections in a fifteen minute listening time on each of three consecutive days.

L = Listening with Eyes and Brain
When listening and reading along to an oral story at Student's social cognitive level, Student will make text connections (i.e., text-to-text, text-to-self, text-to-world) that demonstrate thinking with eyes and brain (e.g., "I see…which makes me think of…" or "That makes me wonder…"), improving listening with eyes and brain from X out of 5 to 4 out of 5 in each session on three consecutive data days.

A = Abstract/Inferential Language
When listening and reading along to an oral story at Student's social cognitive level, Student will make text connections (i.e., text-to-text,

text-to-self, text-to-world) that demonstrate inferencing (e.g., "That character probably won't do that because..."), improving abstract and inferential language skills from X out of 5 to 4 out of 5 in each session on three consecutive data days.

U = Understanding Perspective

When listening and reading along to an oral story at Student's social cognitive level, Student will make text connections (i.e., text-to-text, text-to-self, text-to-world) that demonstrate understanding perspective (e.g., "He felt/thought the same/different in..." or "I have felt/thought the same/different..."), improving from X out of 5 to 4 out of 5 in each session on three consecutive data days.

G = Gestalt Processing/Getting the Big Picture

When listening and reading along to an oral story at Student's social cognitive level, Student will make text connections (i.e., text-to-text, text-to-self, text-to-world) that demonstrate gestalt processing (e.g., "The other chapter/book was the same/different because..." or answers "What other real or written stories have the same main idea" questioning), improving from X out of 5 to 4 out of 5 in each session on three consecutive data days.

H = Humor and Human Relatedness

When listening and reading along to an oral story at Student's social cognitive level, Student will make text connections (i.e., text-to-text, text-to-self, text-to-world) that demonstrate humor and human relatedness (e.g., "She thinks/feels...which is the same/different as..." or "I heard a joke like that..."), improving from X out of 5 to 4 out of 5 in each session on three consecutive data days.

Reading Comprehension Strategy:
Goal Ideas for Visualizing

Thinking with Eyes

When listening and reading along to an oral story at Student's social cognitive level, Student will comment about visualizations that demonstrate thinking with eyes (e.g., "In my head picture, I see..." or "When I hear that, I see...in my head picture"), improving from X out of 5 to 4 out of 5 in each session on three consecutive data days.

Body in the Group

When listening and reading along to an oral story at Student's social cognitive level, Student will keep his or her body in the group while visualizing the story, improving from requiring X reminders in five minutes to return his or her body to group to requiring no reminders every five minutes for a total of fifteen minutes listening time on three consecutive data days.

Keeping Brain in the Group

When listening and reading along to an oral story at Student's social cognitive level, Student will demonstrate he or she is keeping his or her brain in the group by commenting about visualizations (e.g., "In my head picture, I see…" or "When I hear that, I see…in my head picture"), improving from X out of 5 to 4 out of 5 in each session on three consecutive data days.

I = Initiation of Language

When listening and reading along to an oral story at Student's social cognitive level, Student will initiate a question or comment about visualizations (e.g., "I see…in my head picture" or "What does…look like in your head picture?") in a group setting, improving initiation of language from initiating X comments to initiating X comments in a fifteen minute listening time on each of three consecutive days.

L = Listening with Eyes and Brain

When listening and reading along to an oral story at Student's social cognitive level, Student will comment about visualizations that demonstrate thinking with eyes and brain (e.g., "In my head picture, I see…" or "When I hear that, I see…in my head picture"), improving listening with eyes and brain from X out of 5 to 4 out of 5 in each session on three consecutive data days.

A = Abstract/Inferential Language

When listening and reading along to an oral story at Student's social cognitive level, Student will comment about visualizations that demonstrate inferencing (e.g., "I can see…in my head picture because…" or "Because he… I see… in my head picture"), improving abstract and inferential language skills from X out of 5 to 4 out of 5 in each session on three consecutive data days.

U = Understanding Perspective

When listening and reading along to an oral story at Student's social cognitive level, Student will comment about visualizations that demonstrate understanding perspective (e.g., "She probably had... in her head picture" or "He was thinking..."), improving from X out of 5 to 4 out of 5 in each session on three consecutive data days.

G = Gestalt Processing/Getting the Big Picture

When listening and reading along to an oral story at Student's social cognitive level, Student will comment about visualizations that demonstrate gestalt processing (e.g., describes final "head picture" at the end of a story or answers "How did that change your head picture" questioning), improving from X out of 5 to 4 out of 5 in each session on three consecutive data days.

H = Humor and Human Relatedness

When listening and reading along to an oral story at Student's social cognitive level, Student will comment about visualizations that demonstrate humor and human relatedness (e.g., "I see them... in my head picture" or "When they... I see... in my head picture"), improving from X out of 5 to 4 out of 5 in each session on three consecutive data days.

Reading Comprehension Strategy:
Goal Ideas for Inferencing

Expected/Unexpected Behavior

When listening and reading along to an oral story at Student's social cognitive level, Student will make inferences about expected and unexpected behaviors by identifying them in stories, improving from X out of 5 to 4 out of 5 in each session on three consecutive data days.

The Social Fake

When listening and reading along to an oral story at Student's social cognitive level, Student will identify in the story where characters are engaged in "The Social Fake" in order to have socially-acceptable behavior, improving from X out of 5 to 4 out of 5 in each session on three consecutive data days.

Whopping Topic Change
When listening and reading along to an oral story at Student's social cognitive level, Student will make inferences about the impact of on- and off-topic commenting in conversation by identifying when it happens in stories, improving from X out of 5 to 4 out of 5 in each session on three consecutive data days.

I = Initiation of Language
When listening and reading along to an oral story at Student's social cognitive level, Student will initiate a question or comment about inferencing (e.g., "I think that means…" or "Why did she do…?") in a group setting, improving initiation of language from initiating X comments in five minutes to initiating X comments in a fifteen minute listening time on each of three consecutive days.

L = Listening with Eyes and Brain
When listening and reading along to an oral story at Student's social cognitive level, Student will make an inference that demonstrates thinking with eyes and brain (e.g., "I think these are…because I see…" or "I think there is…because I know that…"), improving listening with eyes and brain from X out of 5 to 4 out of 5 in each session on three consecutive data days.

A = Abstract/Inferential Language
When listening and reading along to an oral story at Student's social cognitive level, Student will make an inference (e.g., "I think… because…" or "Because he… I think…"), improving abstract and inferential language skills from X out of 5 to 4 out of 5 in each session on three consecutive data days.

U = Understanding Perspective
When listening and reading along to an oral story at Student's social cognitive level, Student will make an inference that demonstrates understanding perspective (e.g., "She probably thinks/feels… because…" or "He was thinking/feeling…"), improving from X out of 5 to 4 out of 5 in each session on three consecutive data days.

G = Gestalt Processing/Getting the Big Picture
When listening and reading along to an oral story at Student's social

cognitive level, Student will make an inference that demonstrates gestalt processing (e.g., "The whole story is saying…" or answers "What's the main idea" questioning), improving from X out of 5 to 4 out of 5 in each session on three consecutive data days.

H = Humor and Human Relatedness

When listening and reading along to an oral story at Student's social cognitive level, Student will make an inference that demonstrates humor and human relatedness (e.g., "I think they… because…" or "It's funny because…"), improving from X out of 5 to 4 out of 5 in each session on three consecutive data days.

Reading Comprehension Strategy: Goal Ideas for Synthesizing/Summarizing

Boring Moments

When listening and reading along to an oral story at Student's social cognitive level, Student will do the Social Fake during a discussion that doesn't interest Student by participating in summarizing activities, improving from initiating X relevant comments in five minutes to initiating X relevant comments in a fifteen minute listening period on each of three consecutive days.

Flexible Brain

When listening and reading along to an oral story at Student's social cognitive level, Student will demonstrate knowledge of a flexible brain by identifying examples of it and occurrences that are not examples in stories during summarizing, improving from X out of 5 to 4 out of 5 in each session on three consecutive data days.

Rubber Chicken Moments

When listening and reading along to an oral story at Student's social cognitive level, Student will demonstrate knowledge of social mishaps by identifying them in stories during summarizing, improving from X out of 5 to 4 out of 5 in each session on three consecutive data days.

I = Initiation of Language

When listening and reading along to an oral story at Student's social cognitive level, Student will initiate a question or comment demonstrating summarizing (e.g., "In this story…" or "What happened when…?") in a group setting, improving initiation of language from initiating X comments in five minutes to initiating an average of X comments every five minutes for a total of fifteen minutes listening time on three consecutive data days.

L = Listening with Eyes and Brain

When listening and reading along to an oral story at Student's social cognitive level, Student will make summarizing comments that demonstrate thinking with eyes and brain (e.g., "I remember they…" or "The story was…"), improving listening with eyes and brain from X out of 5 to 4 out of 5 in each session on three consecutive data days.

A = Abstract/Inferential Language

When listening and reading along to an oral story at Student's social cognitive level, Student will make summarizing comments that demonstrate inferencing (e.g., "I think… because…" or "Because she… I think…"), improving abstract and inferential language skills from X out of 5 to 4 out of 5 in each session on three consecutive data days.

U = Understanding Perspective

When listening and reading along to an oral story at Student's social cognitive level, Student will make summarizing comments that demonstrate understanding perspective (e.g., "He probably thinks/feels… because…" or "She was thinking/feeling…"), improving from X out of 5 to 4 out of 5 in each session on three consecutive data days.

G = Gestalt Processing/Getting the Big Picture

When listening and reading along to an oral story at Student's social cognitive level, Student will make summarizing comments that demonstrate gestalt processing (e.g., "The whole story is saying…" or answers "What happened in this story" questioning), improving from X out of 5 to 4 out of 5 in each session on three consecutive data days.

H = Humor and Human Relatedness

When listening and reading along to an oral story at Student's social cognitive level, Student will make summarizing comments that demonstrate humor and human relatedness (e.g., "I think they... because...," "It's funny because...," or "They learned that..."), improving from X out of 5 to 4 out of 5 in each session on three consecutive data days.

Reading Comprehension Strategy: Goal Ideas for Building on Prior Knowledge

Good and Uncomfortable Thoughts
When listening and reading along to an oral story at Student's social cognitive level, Student will demonstrate knowledge of good and uncomfortable thoughts by building on prior knowledge (e.g., identify how a situation or character had previously created good or uncomfortable thoughts), improving from X out of 5 to 4 out of 5 in each session on three consecutive data days.

Body in the Group
When listening and reading along to an oral story at Student's social cognitive level, Student will keep his or her body in the group while participating in a discussion about building on prior knowledge, from requiring X reminders in five minutes to return body to group to requiring no reminders every five minutes for a total of fifteen minutes listening time on three consecutive data days.

People (or Friend) Files
When listening and reading along to an oral story at Student's social cognitive level, Student will build on prior knowledge that demonstrates knowledge of friend files (e.g., "Jason knows that Sally doesn't like peanuts because he learned that in the last chapter"), improving from X out of 5 to 4 out of 5 in each session on three consecutive data days.

I = Initiation of Language
When listening and reading along to an oral story at Student's social cognitive level, Student will initiate a question or comment demonstrating prior knowledge (e.g., "Previously..., and now..." or "What did it mean in the other story when...?") in a group setting, improving initiation of language from initiating X comments to initiating X comments in a fifteen minute listening time on each of three consecutive days.

L = Listening with Eyes and Brain

When listening and reading along to an oral story at Student's social cognitive level, Student will use prior knowledge to demonstrate thinking with eyes and brain (e.g., "I remember they..." or "I remember seeing... "), improving listening with eyes and brain from X out of 5 to 4 out of 5 in each session on three consecutive data days.

A = Abstract/Inferential Language

When listening and reading along to an oral story at Student's social cognitive level, Student will use prior knowledge to demonstrate inferencing (e.g., "I think... because..." or "Because he... I think..."), improving abstract and inferential language skills from X out of 5 to 4 out of 5 in each session on three consecutive data days.

U = Understanding Perspective

When listening and reading along to an oral story at Student's social cognitive level, Student will use prior knowledge to demonstrate understanding perspective (e.g., "I already know she..., so she probably thinks/feels..." or "He was thinking/feeling..."), improving from X out of 5 to 4 out of 5 in each session on three consecutive data days.

G = Gestalt Processing/Getting the Big Picture

When listening and reading along to an oral story at Student's social cognitive level, Student will use prior knowledge to demonstrate gestalt processing (e.g., "I already knew..., and now I know... from this story" or "The other book..."), improving from X out of 5 to 4 out of 5 in each session on three consecutive data days.

H = Humor and Human Relatedness

When listening and reading along to an oral story at Student's social cognitive level, Student will use prior knowledge to demonstrate humor and human relatedness (e.g., "I think they... because I know they... previously" or "It's funny because..."), improving from X out of 5 to 4 out of 5 in each session on three consecutive data days.

Reading Comprehension Strategy:
Goal Ideas for Sequencing

Size of Problems

When listening and reading along to an oral story at Student's social cognitive level, Student will demonstrate knowledge of size of problems during sequencing activities by identifying sizes of problems encountered in stories, improving from X out of 5 to 4 out of 5 in each session on three consecutive data days.

Whopping Topic Change

When listening and reading along to an oral story at Student's social cognitive level, Student will demonstrate knowledge of the impact of on- and off-topic commenting in conversation by identifying when it happens in stories during sequencing activities, improving from X out of 5 to 4 out of 5 in each session on three consecutive data days.

Thinking About You/Just Me

When listening and reading along to an oral story at Student's social cognitive level, Student will demonstrate Thinking About You/Just Me during sequencing activities (e.g., "She was a Just Me when..." or "After that, he became a Thinking About You person"), improving from X out of 5 to 4 out of 5 in each session on three consecutive data days.

I = Initiation of Language

When listening and reading along to an oral story at Student's social cognitive level, Student will initiate a question or comment demonstrating sequencing (e.g., "First, they..., then they..." or "What happened after...?") in a group setting, improving initiation of language from initiating X comments in five minutes to initiating an average of X comments every five minutes for a total of fifteen minutes listening time on three consecutive data days.

L = Listening with Eyes and Brain

When listening and reading along to an oral story at Student's social cognitive level, Student will make sequencing comments that demonstrate thinking with eyes and brain (e.g., "I remember they... and then..." or "Earlier, there was... "), improving listening with eyes and brain from X out of 5 to 4 out of 5 in each session on three consecutive data days.

A = Abstract/Inferential Language

When listening and reading along to an oral story at Student's social cognitive level, Student will make sequencing comments that demonstrate inferencing (e.g., "She previously..., so I think she means..." or "There was... so now I think it means..."), improving abstract and inferential language skills from X out of 5 to 4 out of 5 in each session on three consecutive data days.

U = Understanding Perspective

When listening and reading along to an oral story at Student's social cognitive level, Student will make sequencing comments that demonstrate understanding perspective (e.g., "He used to, so he probably thinks/feels..." or "She was thinking/feeling..., so now..."), improving from X out of 5 to 4 out of 5 in each session on three consecutive data days.

G = Gestalt Processing/Getting the Big Picture

When listening and reading along to an oral story at Student's social cognitive level, Student will make sequencing comments that demonstrate gestalt processing (e.g., "First, ..., then..., so I think the meaning is..." or answers "What happened in this story" questioning), improving from X out of 5 to 4 out of 5 in each session on three consecutive data days.

H = Humor and Human Relatedness

When listening and reading along to an oral story at Student's social cognitive level, Student will make sequencing comments that demonstrate humor and human relatedness (e.g., "Previously, they..., so now they think/feel...," "It's funny because...," or "They learned... when..."), improving from X out of 5 to 4 out of 5 in each session on three consecutive data days.

References

Suggested Books for Book Chats

Archambault, J. (2004). *Boom chicka rock*. New York: Philomel.

Arnold, T. (2001). *More parts*. New York: Dial Books for Young Readers.

Baker, J. (2006). *The social skills picture book for high school and beyond*. Arlington, TX: Future Horizons Inc.

Bang, M. (1999). *When Sophie gets angry—really, really angry....* New York: The Blue Sky Press.

Binkow, H. (2006.) *Howard B. Wigglebottom learns to listen*. Minneapolis, MN: Lerner Publishing Group.

Blumenthal, D. (1996). *The chocolate-covered-cookie tantrum*. New York: Clarion Books.

Bottner, B. (1992). *Bootsie Barker bites*. New York: G.P. Putnam's Sons.

Breathed, B. (1995). *A wish for wings that work: An opus Christmas story*. New York: Little, Brown Books for Young Readers.

Breathed, B. (2003). *Edwurd Fudwupper fibbed big*. New York: Little, Brown Books for Young Readers.

Breathed, B. (2007). *Mars needs moms!* New York: Philomel Books.

Brown, L.K., & Brown, M. (1998). *How to be a friend: A guide to making friends and keeping them*. Boston: Little, Brown.

Carlson, N. (2006). *First grade, here I come!* New York: Viking.

Carlson, N. (1994). *How to lose all your friends*. New York: Penguin Books.

Carlson, N. (2003). *It's not my fault!* Minneapolis: Carolrhoda Books, Inc.

Carlson, N. (1996). *Sit still!* New York: Puffin Books.

Cook, J. (2005). *A bad case of tattle tongue*. Chattanooga, TN: National Center for Youth Issues.

Cook, J. (2010 reprint). *I am a booger...treat me with respect!* Chattanooga, TN: National Center for Youth Issues.

Cook, J. (2006). *My mouth is a volcano!* Chattanooga, TN: National Center for Youth Issues.

Cook, J. (2007). *Personal space camp.* Chattanooga, TN: National Center for Youth Issues.

Cooke, K. (first U.S. edition, 2003). *The terrible underpants.* New York: Hyperion Books for Children.

Cooper, B., & Widdows, N. (2008). *The social success workbook for teens.* Oakland, CA: Instant Help Books.

Diesen, D. (2008). *The pout-pout fish.* New York: Farrar, Straus and Giroux.

Dr. Seuss [pseud.]. (1957). *The cat in the hat.* Boston: Houghton Mifflin.

Eastman, P.D. (1960). *Are you my mother?* New York: Random House Books for Young Readers.

Elliott, L. M., & Munsinger, L. (2005). *Hunter's best friend at school.* New York: Katherine Tegen Books.

Emberley, E., & Miranda, A. (1997). *Glad monster, sad monster.* New York: LB Kids.

Emberley, E. (1992). *Go away, big green monster!* New York: Little, Brown and Company.

Epstein, R. (2009). *The worst-case scenario survival handbook: middle school.* San Francisco: Chronicle Books LLC.

Fearnley, J. (2004). *Watch out!* Somerville, MA: Candlewick Press.

Gravett, E. (2009). *The odd egg.* New York: Simon and Schuster Books for Young Readers.

Grossman, B. (1995). *The banging book.* New York, NY: HarperCollins Children's Books.

Hargreaves, R. (2000). *Mr. Daydream.* New York: Price, Stern, Sloan.

Hargreaves, R. (1997). *Mr. Funny.* New York: Price, Stern, Sloan.

Hargreaves, R. (1999). *Mr. Grumpy.* New York: Price, Stern, Sloan.

Hargreaves, R. (2011 reprint). *Little Miss Chatterbox.* New York: Price, Stern, Sloan.

Horvath, D. (2007). *Bossy bear.* New York: Hyperion Books for Children.

Huebner, D. (2006). *What to do when you worry too much: A kid's guide to overcoming anxiety.* Washington, DC: Magination Press. Other what to do guides, such as *What to do when your brain gets stuck: A kid's guide to overcoming OCD,* by the same author are also recommended.

Johnson, A. (2005). *That's not funny!* New York: Bloomsbury USA Children's Books.

Kinney, J. (2007). *Diary of a wimpy kid: A novel in cartoons.* New York: Amulet Books. Other books are also available in this series.

Lehman, B. (2004). *The red book.* Boston: Houghton Mifflin Company.

Lionni, L. (1986, first Dragonfly Books edition 1996). *It's mine!* New York: Dragonfly Books published by Alfred A. Knopf, Inc.

Lionni, L. (2007). *Tico and the golden wings.* New York: Knopf Books for Young Readers.

Luck, D. (2005). *We listen...we don't interrupt.* Wiltshire, Great Britain: Positive Press.

Madrigal, S., & Winner, M.G. (2009). *Superflex takes on Glassman and the team of Unthinkables.* San Jose, CA: Think Social Publishing, Inc.

Madrigal, S. (2008). *Superflex takes on Rock Brain and the team of Unthinkables.* San Jose, CA: Think Social Publishing, Inc.

Martin Jr., B., & Archambault, J. (2000). *Chicka chicka boom boom.* New York: Beach Lane Publishing.

MacLennan, C. (2007). *Chicky chicky chook chook.* Farringdon, London: Boxer Books.

Mayer, M. (2000). *I was so mad.* New York: Random House Books for Young Readers.

Mayer, M. (2001). *Just grandma and me.* New York: Random House Books for Young Readers.

Mayer, M. (2001). *Just me and my dad.* New York: Random House Books for Young Readers.

Mayer, M. (2001). *Just me and my mom.* New York: Random House Books for Young Readers.

Mayer, M. (2001). *Just my friend and me.* New York: Random House Books for Young Readers.

Mayer, M. (1987). *There's an alligator under my bed.* New York: Dial Books for Young Readers.

Meiners, C.J. (2004). *Join in and play.* Minneapolis: Free Spirit Publishing Inc.

Montgomery, R.A. (2007). *Your very own robot.* Waitsfield, VT: Chooseco.

Mundy, M. (2010). *Mad isn't bad: A child's book about anger.* Melnrad, IN: Abbey Press.

Numeroff, L. (1985). *If you give a mouse a cookie.* New York: HarperCollins Publishers.

Numeroff, L. (2008). *Beatrice doesn't want to.* Somerville, MA: Candlewick Press.

O'Neill, A. (2002). *The recess queen.* New York: Scholastic.

Osborne, M.P. (2001). *Earthquake in the early morning.* New York: Random House Books for Young Readers.

Packer, A.J. (2004). *The how rude! handbook of friendship & dating manners for teens: Surviving the social scene.* Minneapolis: Free Spirit Publishing Inc. There are also other *How Rude!* handbooks by the same author.

Ransom, J.F. (2005). *Don't squeal unless it's a big deal: A tale of tattletales.* Washington, DC: Magination Press.

Roland, T. (1997). *Come down now, flying cow!* New York: Random House Books for Young Readers.

Rowling, J.K. (1998). *Harry Potter and the sorcerer's stone.* New York: Scholastic.

Sachar, L. (2004). *Wayside School boxed set: Wayside School gets a little stranger, Wayside School is falling down, Sideway Stories from Wayside School.* New York: HarperCollins.

Schneider, C. (2006). *I'm bored!* New York: Houghton Mifflin Company.

Shannon, D. (1998). *No, David!* New York: The Blue Sky Press.

Sherry, K. (2007). *I'm the biggest thing in the ocean.* New York: Dial Books for Young Readers.

Silverstein, S. (1964, 35th anniversary edition 1999). *The giving tree.* New York: HarperCollins.

Silverstein, S. (1981). *The missing piece meets the big o.* New York: HarperCollins.

Silverstein, S. (1961). *Uncle Shelby's abz book: A primer for adults only.* New York: Simon & Schuster, Inc.

Slonim, D. (2005). *He came with the couch.* San Francisco: Chronicle Books.

Stover, J.A. (1990). *If everybody did.* Greenville, SC: JourneyForth.

Tankard, J. (2007). *Grumpy bird.* New York: Scholastic.

Tunis, S.L. (2004). *Why can't Jimmy sit still?* Far Hills, NY: New Horizon Press.

Verdick, E., & Lisovskis, M. (2003). *How to take the grrr out of anger.* Minneapolis, MN: Free Spirit Publishing Inc.

Viorst, J. (1972). *Alexander and the terrible, horrible, no good, very bad day.* New York: Atheneum.

Watt, M. (2008). *Scaredy squirrel.* Toronto, Canada: Kids Can Press, Ltd. There are other books in this series by the same author.

Willems, M. (2003). *Don't let the pigeon drive the bus!* New York: Hyperion Books for Children.

Wood, A. (1984). *The napping house.* San Diego, CA: Harcourt Brace Jovanovich.

Wood, A. (1992). *Silly Sally.* San Diego, CA: Harcourt Brace Jovanovich.

Bibliography

Dyslexia and hyperlexia: Diagnosis and management of developmental reading disabilities. Dordrecht, ND: Kluwer Academic Publishers.

Anderson, R.C. & Pearson, P.D. (1984). A schemata-theoretic view of basic processes in reading comprehension. In P.D. Pearson, R. Barr, M. Kamil, & P. Mosenthal (Eds.), *Handbook of reading research* (pp. 255-291). New York: Longman.

Åsberg, J. (2009). Literacy and comprehension in school-aged children: Studies on autism and other developmental disabilities [Elektronisk resurs]. Intellecta Infolog AB. Available on the Internet: http://hdl.handle.net/2077/21063

Barnes, M.A., Dennis, M., & Haefele-Kalvaitis, J. (1996). The effects of knowledge availability and knowledge accessibility on coherence and elaborative inferencing in children from six to fifteen years of age. *Journal of Experimental Child Psychology, 61,* 216–241.

Baron-Cohen, S., Leslie, A. M., & Frith, U. (1985). Does the autistic child have a "theory of mind"? *Cognition, 21,* 37–46.

Bishop, D.V.M. (1997). *Uncommon understanding.* Hove, UK: Psychology Press.

Bruner, J. (1986). *Actual minds, possible worlds.* Cambridge, MA: Harvard University Press.

Burd, L., & Kerbeshian, J. (1985). Hyperlexia and a variant of hypergraphia. *Perceptual and Motor Skills,* 50, 940–942.

Burd, L., Kerbeshian, J., Fisher, W. (1985). Inquiry into the incidence of hyperlexia in a statewide population of children with pervasive developmental disorder. *Psychological Reports,* 57, 236–238.

Cain, J., & Oakhill, J. (2007). Introduction to comprehension development. In Cain, J. & Oakhill, J. (Eds.), *Children's Comprehension Problems in Oral and Written Language* (pp. 3–40). New York, NY: Guilford Press.

Cain, K., & Oakhill, J. V. (1999). Inference ability and its relation to comprehension failure in young children. *Reading and Writing,* 11, 489–503.

Cain, K., Oakhill, J.V., & Lemmon, K. (2004). Individual differences in the inference of word meanings from context: the influence of reading comprehension, vocabulary knowledge, and memory capacity. *Journal of Educational Psychology,* 96, 671–681.

Carr E., Dewitz, P., & Patberg, J. (1989). Using cloze for inference training with expository text. *The Reading Teacher,* 42(6), 380–385.

Chall, J.S. (1967). *Learning to read: The great debate.* New York: McGraw Hill.

Chall, J.S. (1996). *Stages of reading development, 2nd edition.* Orlando, FL: Harcourt Brace & Company.

Courchesne E., Townsend, J., Akshoomoff, N., Saitoh, O., Yeung-Courchesne, R., Lincoln, A., James, H., Haas, R., Schreibman, L., & Lau, L. (1994). Impairment in shifting attention in autistic and cerebellar patients. *Behavioral Neuroscience,* 108(5), 848–865.

Crooke, P., Hendrix, R., & Rachman, J. (2007). Brief report: measuring the effectiveness of teaching Social Thinking to children with Asperger Syndrome (AS) and high functioning autism (HFA). *Journal of Autism and Developmental Disorders.*

Cunningham, A.E. (2005). Vocabulary growth through independent reading and reading aloud to children. In E.H. Hiebert & M.L. Kamil (Eds.), *Teaching and learning vocabulary: Bringing research to practice* (pp. 45-68).

Mahwah, NJ: Erlbaum.

de C. Hamilton, A.F., Brindley, R., & Frith, U. (2007). Imitation and action understanding in autistic spectrum disorders: How valid is the hypothesis of a deficit in the mirror neuron system? Neuropsychologia, 45, 1859–1868.

Franco, F. (1997). The development of meaning in infancy: early communication and social understanding. In S. Hala, *The development of social cognition* (pp. 95–146). United Kingdom: Psychology Press.

Garfield, J., Peterson, C., & Perry, T. (2001). Social cognition, language acquisition and the development of the theory of mind. *Mind and Language,* 16(5), 494–541.

Garton, A., & Pratt, C. (1998). *Learning to be literate: The development of spoken and written language* (2nd ed.). Oxford, UK: Blackwell.

Goldstein, G., Minshew, N., & Siegel, D. (1994). Age differences in academic achievement in high-functioning autistic individuals. *Journal of Clinical and Experimental Neuropsychology,* 16(5), 671–680.

Gough, P.B., & Tunmer, W.E. (1986). Decoding, reading, and reading disability. *Remedial and Special Education,* 7(1), 6–10.

Greeno, J. G., Collins, A. M., & Resnick, L. B. (1996). Cognition and learning. In D. Berliner and R. Calfee (Eds.), *Handbook of Educational Psychology* (pp. 15-41). New York: MacMillian.

Grigorenko, E.L., Klin, A., Pauls, D.L., Senft, R., Hooper, C., & Volkmar, F. (2002). A descriptive study of hyperlexia in a clinically referred sample of children with developmental delays. *Journal of Autism and Developmental Disorders,* 32, 3–12.

Happé, F.G.E. (1997). Central coherence and theory of mind in autism: reading homographs in context. *British Journal of Developmental Psychology,* 15, 1–12.

Jensen, A.K. (2006). Reading profile in students with high-functioning autism and hyperlexia. (Unpublished Master's Thesis, University of Washington).

Keene, E., & Zimmermann, S. (2007). *Mosaic of thought, second edition: the power of comprehension strategy instruction.* Portsmouth, NH: Heineman.

Kendeou, P., Lynch, L.S., van den Broek, P., Espin, C., White, M., & Kremerk, K.E. (2006). Developing successful readers: building early narrative comprehension skills through television viewing and listening. *Early Childhood Education Journal*, 33(2), 91–98.

Kendeou, P., van den Broek, P., White, M.J., & Lynch, J. (2007). Comprehension in preschool and early elementary children: Skill development and strategy interventions. In D.S. McNamara (Ed.), *Reading comprehension strategies: Theories, interventions, and technologies*. Mahwah, NJ: Erlbaum.

Kintsch, W. (1998). *Comprehension: a paradigm for cognition*. New York: Cambridge University Press.

LaBerge, D., & Samuels, S.J. (1974). Toward a theory of automatic information processing in reading. *Cognitive Psychology*, 6, 293–323.

Laing, S., & Kamhi, A. (2002). The use of think-aloud protocols to compare inferencing abilities of average and below-average readers. *Journal of Learning Disabilities*, 35, 437–448.

Lee, K., Lui, A., Kan, P., Mak, K., Cheung, P., Cheng, L., & Wong, I. (2009). A case series on the social thinking training of mainstreamed secondary school students with high-functioning autism. *Hong Kong Journal of Mental Health*, 35, 10–17.

McGee, A., & Johnson, H. (2003). The effects of inference training on skilled and less skilled comprehenders. *Educational Psychology*, 23, 49–59.

Minshewa, N., Goldstein, G., Taylor, H., & Siegel, D. (1994). Academic achievement in high functioning autistic individuals. *Journal of Clinical and Experimental Neuropsychology*, 16(2), 261–270.

Moreau, M.R. (2010). It's all about the story! Springfield, MA: MindWing Concepts, Inc.

Nation, K., Clarke, P., Wright, B., & Williams, C. (2006). Patterns of reading ability in children with autism spectrum disorders. *Journal of Autism and Developmental Disorders*, 36, 911–919.

National Reading Panel (NRP). (2000). *Teaching children to read: An evidence-based assessment of the scientific research literature on reading and its implications for reading instruction: Reports of the subgroups*. Bethesda, MD: NICHD.

New England Common Assessment Program (NECAP). (n.d.). Retrieved March 1, 2010, from Department of Education, State of Main website: http://www.maine.gov/education/necap/march2005_reading2-5gles.v18.2.pdf.

No Child Left Behind Act of 2001. Pub. L. No. 107-110. 115 Stat. 1425 (2002). Retrieved March 1, 2010, from U.S. Department of Education website: http://www2.ed.gov/policy/elsec/leg/esea02/107-110.pdf.

Oakhill, J. V., Cain, K., & Bryan, P. (2003). The dissociation of word reading and text comprehension: evidence from component skills. *Language and Cognitive Processes, 18,* 443–468.

Oakhill, J., Yuill, N., & Parkin, A. (1986). On the nature of the difference between skilled and less-skilled comprehenders. *Journal of Research in Reading, 9,* 80–91.

Online Grade Level Standards and Resources Reading. (n.d.). Retrieved March 1, 2010, from Washington State Office of Superintendent of Public Instruction website: http://standards.ospi.k12.wa.us/ComponentWithGLEs.aspx?subject=1,GLE&gl=4&ea=2&co=6.

Paris, S.G., & Hamilton, E.E. (2009). The development of children's reading comprehension. In *Handbook of Research on Reading Comprehension* (pp. 32-53). New York, NY: Taylor & Francis.

Paris, S.G., & Stahl, S.A. (2005). *Children's reading comprehension and assessment.* Mahwah, NJ: Erlbaum.

Pelletier, J., & Astington, J. (2004). Action, consciousness and theory of mind: children's ability to coordinate story characters' actions and thoughts. Early Education & Development, 15(1), 5–22.

Perfetti, C.A. (1994). Psycholinguistics and reading ability. In M.A. Gernsbacher (Ed.), *Handbook of psycholinguistics* (pp. 849-894). San Diego: Academic Press.

Plaisted, K., Swettenham, J., & Rees, L. (1999). Children with autism show local precedence in a divided attention task and global precedence in a selective attention task. *Journal of Child Psychology and Psychiatry,* 40(5), 733–742.

Pressley, M., & Afflerbach, P. (1995). *Verbal protocols of reading: The nature of constructively responsive reading.* Hillsdale, NJ: Erlbaum.

Rathvon, N. (2004). *Early reading assessment: A practitioner's handbook.* New York: Guilford Press.

Reid, J.F. (1970). Sentence structure in reading primers. *Research in Education,* 3, 23–37.

Reid, J.F. (1983). Into print: reading and language growth. In M. Donaldson, R. Grief, & C. Pratt (Eds.), *Early childhood development and education* (pp. 151-165). Oxford, UK: Basil Blackwell.

Reutzel, D. R., & Hollingsworth, P. M. (1988). Getting a grip on inferential comprehension: a procedure for teaching selected inference types. *Reading Horizons,* 29, 71–78.

Rogers, K., Dziobek, I., Hassenstab, J., Wolf, O.T., & Convit, A. Who cares? Revisiting empathy in Asperger's syndrome. *J Autism Dev Disord.* 2007 Apr, 37(4), 709–15.

Rumelhart, D.E. (1994). Toward an interactive model of reading. In R.B. Ruddell, M. Rapp-Ruddell, & H. Singer (Eds.), *Theoretical models of processes of reading, 4th ed.* (pp. 864–894). Newark, DE: International Reading Association.

Selman, R.L. (1999). The development of social-cognitive understanding: a guide to education and clinical practice. In J. Santrock, *Life-span development* (pp. 313). Boston: McGraw-Hill Publishing.

Shah, A., & Frith, U. (1993). Why do autistic individuals show superior performance on the block design task? *Journal of Child Psychology and Psychiatry,* 34(8), 1351–1364.

Silberberg, N., & Silberberg, M. (1967). Hyperlexia: specific word recognition skills in young children. *Exceptional Children,* 34, 41–42.

Snowling, M., & Frith, U. (1986). Comprehension in "hyperlexic" readers. *Journal of Experimental Child Psychology,* 42, 392–415.

Stahl, S.A., & Hiebert, E.H. (2005). The "word factors": A problem for reading comprehension assessments. In S.G. Paris & S.A. Stahl (Eds.), *Current issues in reading comprehension and assessment* (pp. 161–186). Mahwah, NJ: Erlbaum.

Stahl, S.A., Kuhn, M.R., & Pickle, J.M. (1999). An educational model of assessment and targeted instruction for children with reading problems. In D. Evenson & P. Mosenthal (Eds.), *Reconsidering the role of the reading clinic in a new age of literacy* (pp. 249–272). Greenwich, CT: JAI Press.

Texas essential knowledge and skills for English Language Arts and Reading. (n.d.). Retrieved March 1, 2010, from Texas Education Agency website: http://ritter.tea.state.tx.us/rules/tac/chapter110/ch110a.html.

Tovani, C. (2000). *I read it, but I don't get it: comprehension strategies for adolescent readers.* Portland, ME: Stenhouse Publishers.

Trabasso, T., & Nickels, M. (1992). The development of goal plans of action in the narration of a picture story. *Discourse Processes, 15,* 249–275.

U.S. Department of Education. (1994). Improving America's Schools Act of 1994. Retrieved March 1, 2010, from U.S. Department of Education website: http://www2.ed.gov/legislation/ESEA/toc.html.

U.S. Department of Education. (April 1983). A nation at risk. Retrieved March 1, 2010, from U.S. Department of Education website: http://www.ed.gov/pubs/NatAtRisk/risk.html.

Udvari-Solner, A., & Kluth, P. (2007). *Joyful learning.* Thousand Oaks, CA: Corwin Press.

van den Broek, P., Kendeou, P., Kremer, K., Lynch, J.S., Butler, J., White, M.J., et al. (2005). Assessment of comprehension abilities in young children. In S.G. Paris & S.A. Stahl (Eds.), *Children's reading comprehension and assessment* (pp. 107–130). Mahah, NJ: Erlbaum.

Van Dijk, T. A., & Kintsch, W. (1983). *Strategies of discourse comprehension.* New York: Academic.

Vidal-Abarca, E., Martínez, G., & Gilabert, R. (2000). Two procedures to improve instructional text: Effects on memory and learning. *Journal of Educational Psychology, 92*(1), 107–116.

Wahlberg, T., & Magliano, J. (2004). The ability of high function individuals with autism to comprehend written discourse. *Discourse Processes, 38*(1), 119–144.

Walden, T., & Ogan, T. (1988). The development of social referencing. *Child Development, 59,* 1230–1240.

Westby, C. (2004). A language perspective on executive functioning, metacognition, and self-regulation in reading. In C.A. Stone, E. Sillman, B. Ehren, & K. Appel (Eds.), *Handbook* of language and literacy: development and disorders (pp. 398–418). New York: The Guilford Press.

Westby, C. (7/28/2008). Language impairments & social-emotional communicative competence. Retrieved from http://www.speechpathology.com/articles/article_detail.asp?article_id=345.

Winner, M.G. (2000). *Inside out: what makes a person with social cognitive deficits tick?* San Jose, CA: Think Social Publishing.

Winner, M.G. (2008). *Think social! A social thinking curriculum for school-age students for teaching social thinking and related skills to students with high functioning autism, PDD-NOS, Asperger's Syndrome, Nonverbal Learning Disability, ADHD.* San Jose, CA: Think Social Publishing.

Winner, M.G. (2007). *Thinking about you, thinking about me (2nd edition).* San Jose, CA: Think Social Publishing, Inc.

Yuill, N., & Oakhill, J. (1988). Understanding of anaphoric relations in skilled and less skilled comprehenders. *British Journal of Psychology, 79,* 173–186.

About the Author

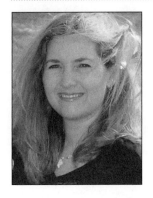

Audra Jensen, a certified Special Education teacher and a Board-Certified Behavior Analyst, got her start as a parent of a child with autism. She has since been interested in the field of reading comprehension and social thinking and how they are interlaced in students with social cognitive disorders. Audra now runs a clinic which provides behavior analytic services and social thinking groups to students with autism and related disorders. She lives in Vancouver, WA with a doting husband, two kids, and two lovable canine companions.

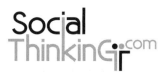

Other products developed by Michelle Garcia Winner
and Social Thinking Publishing

Inside Out: What Makes a Person with Social Cognitive Deficits Tick?

Thinking About You Thinking About Me 2nd Edition

Worksheets for Teaching Social Thinking® and Related Skills

Think Social! A Social Thinking® Curriculum for School Age Students

*Social Behavior Mapping: Connecting Behavior, Emotions
and Consequences Across the Day*
available in English and Spanish

*Sticker Strategies:
Practical Strategies to Encourage Social Thinking and Organization*
2nd Edition

*Strategies for Organization:
Preparing for Homework and the Real World*

Superflex®... A Superhero Social Thinking® Curriculum
(co-authored by Stephanie Madrigal)

Superflex® Takes on Rock Brain and the Team of Unthinkables
(co-authored by Stephanie Madrigal)

Superflex® Takes on Glassman and the Team of Unthinkables
(co-authored by Stephanie Madrigal)

Social Thinking® Across the Home and School Day

You Are a Social Detective!
(co-authored by Pamela Crooke)
available in English, French, and Spanish

*A Politically Incorrect Look at Evidence-Based Practices and Teaching
Social Skills: A literature review and discussion*

*Socially Curious and Curiously Social:
A Social Thinking® Guidebook for Teens and Young Adults*

*Social Fortune or Social Fate
Watch Their Destiny Unfold Based on the Choices They Make*
(co-authored by Pamela Crooke)

*Social Thinking® Worksheets for Tweens and Teens
Learning to Read in Between the Social Lines*

*Social Thinking® at Work: Why Should I Care?
A Guidebook for Understanding and Navigating
the Social Complexities of the Workplace*
(co-authored by Pamela Crooke)

Whole Body Listening Larry at Home!
By Kristen Wilson & Elizabeth Sautter

Whole Body Listening Larry at School!
By Elizabeth Sautter & Kristen Wilson

*We Can Make It Better! Stories©
A Strategy to Motivate and Engage Young Learners
in Social Problem-Solving Through Flexible Stories*
By Elizabeth M. Delsandro

The Zones of Regulation®
A Curriculum Designed to Foster Self-regulation and Emotional Control
By Leah M. Kuypers, MA Ed. OTR/L

Social Thinking® Posters
for the home and classroom

The Zones of Regulation® Poster
for the home and classroom

Superflex® Poster

www.socialthinking.com